간호 영어 회화

English Conversation for Nurses

군자출판사

간호영어회화

クリステイ一ソのレベルアシプ 看護英会話

첫째판 1쇄 인쇄 | 2009년 4월 25일
첫째판 1쇄 발행 | 2009년 4월 30일

옮 긴 이 최정희
발 행 인 장주연
편집디자인 정은진
표지디자인 이지선
발 행 처 군자출판사
등 록 제 4-139호(1991. 6. 24)

본 사 (110-717) 서울특별시 종로구 인의동 112-1 동원회관 BD 6층
Tel. (02) 762-9194/5 Fax. (02) 764-0209
대구지점 Tel. (053) 428-2748 Fax. (053) 428-2749
광주지점 Tel. (062) 228-0252 Fax. (062) 228-0251
부산지점 Tel. (051) 893-8989 Fax. (051) 893-8986

www.koonja.co.kr

* 파본은 교환하여 드립니다.
* 검인은 옮긴이와의 합의 하에 생략합니다.

ISBN 978-89-6278-117-5

정가 18,000원

서문

국제화 시대에 따른 영어회화 능력의 필요성은 간호업무에 있어서도 예외는 아니어서, 간호사들의 해외 진출 및 해외병원의 국내 유치가 활발히 증대되고 있는 추세에 맞추어 해외에서 뿐만 아니라 국내 임상 현장에서도 간호업무에 필요한 영어 회화의 중요성이 커지고 있다.

이 책은 기존 일본의 "クリステイ一ソのレベルアシプ 看護英会話"를 우리 실정에 맞게 번역한 책으로서, 일상생활에서 필요한 기초 회화부터 임상 현장에서 간호업무를 수행할때 필요한 실무적 대화를 비롯 간호사와 환자, 보호자, 의료팀 및 동료 간호사와의 일반회화를 중심으로 구성되어 있으며, 역할극을 통해 각 상황을 설정하고 연습함으로써 효과적으로 도움이 되는 회화 공부를 할 수 있도록 되어 있다. 또한 임상 영어회화에서 자주 쓰이는 의학용어들이 그림과 함께 정리되어 있어 의학용어가 아직 익숙하지 않은 간호학생들에게도 보다 쉽게 의학용어와 임상 영어회화를 배울 수 있는 기회가 될 것으로 생각한다. 이 책을 번역하고 출간되기까지 많은 지원을 아끼지 않으신 군자출판사 관계자 여러분께 감사드리며, 간호 실무 현장에서 고생하시며 열심히 일하시는 간호사분들께 조그마한 도움이라도 드릴 수 있기를 소망한다.

2009. 4

최 정 희

목 차

UNIT 4. Are you suffering from any illnesses?

UNIT 5. You need to have an MRI.

UNIT 6. You' re going to have a baby!

UNIT 7. My baby has a fever.

UNIT 8. Your surgery will be tomorrow at 10 am.

UNIT 9. How are you feeling?

UNIT 10. Are you worried about anything?

한글번역

Transcripts and Answers

UNIT 1

Do you work in the surgical ward?

한글 번역판 참조(115P)

Activity 1: Listening Practice

CD 2

Listen to the conversations and choose the correct answers.

1. What is the woman's last name?
   a) Delores b) Argentina c) Agosto

2. What is the man's phone number?
   a) 02-6299-8614 b) 02-6299-8641 c) 02-6299-8164

3. What is the woman asking the man?
   a) She wants to know his phone number.
   b) She wants to know his occupation.
   c) She wants to know what he is doing now.

4. What does Harvey Jones do?
   a) She's an obstetrician. b) She's a nurse. c) She's a doctor.

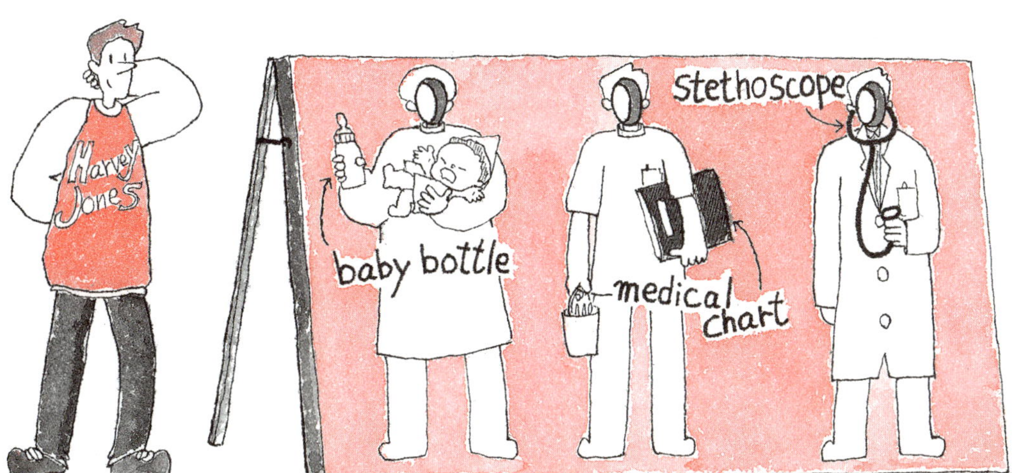

Activity 2: Checkpoint

Emergency English? ~곤란한 상황에서의 영어 회화~
[이탤릭부분을 다른 말로 바꾸어 연습합시다]

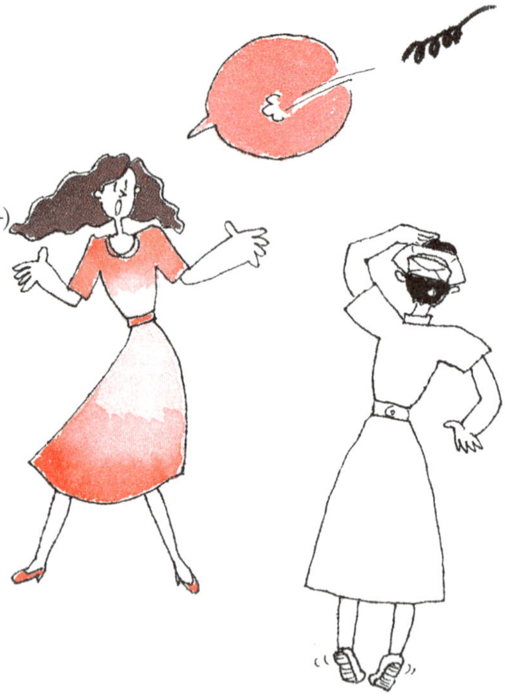

1. 다시 한번 말씀해 주시겠어요?(전문을 되묻는다)
Excuse me?/Pardon?
Could you say that again, please?

2. 13이라고 하셨나요? 30이라고 하셨나요?(일부를 되묻는다)
Did you say thirteen or thirty?

3. 조금 더 천천히 말씀해 주시겠어요?
Could you speak more slowly?

4. 조금 더 크게 말씀해 주시겠어요?
Could you speak more loudly?

5. 죄송합니다. 제가 잘 못 알아 들었습니다.
I' m sorry, I don' t understand.

6. 방사선사는 무슨 일을 하는 사람인가요?
What is the meaning of X-ray technician?

7. 철자를 어떻게 쓰죠?/당신 이름의 성(이름)을 어떻게 쓰죠?
How do you spell that?
How do you spell your family(first) name?

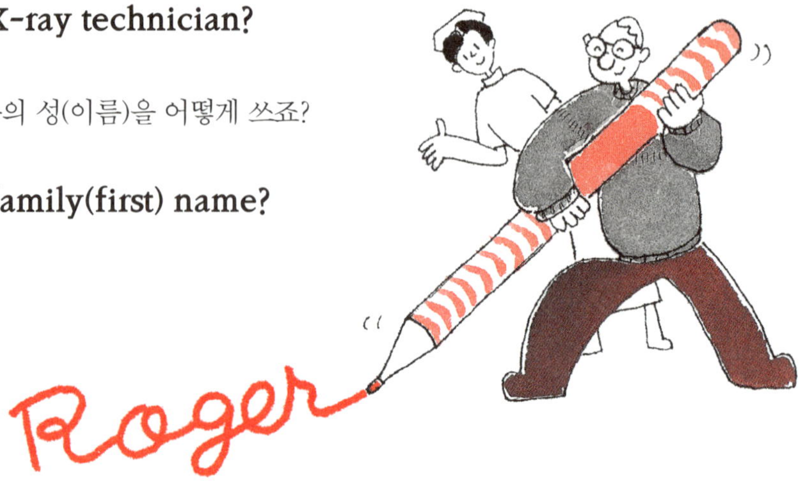

한글 번역판 참조(115P)

초면인사

1. [격식 차린 경우]

Mary: Sam, this is Frank Sawyer. Frank, this is Sam Hernandez.
Sam: How do you do? It' s nice to meet you.
Frank: It' s nice to meet you, too.

2. [친숙한 경우]

Mary: Sam, this is Frank. Frank, this is Sam.
Sam: Hello(hi), It' s nice to meet you.
Frank: Nice to meet you, too.

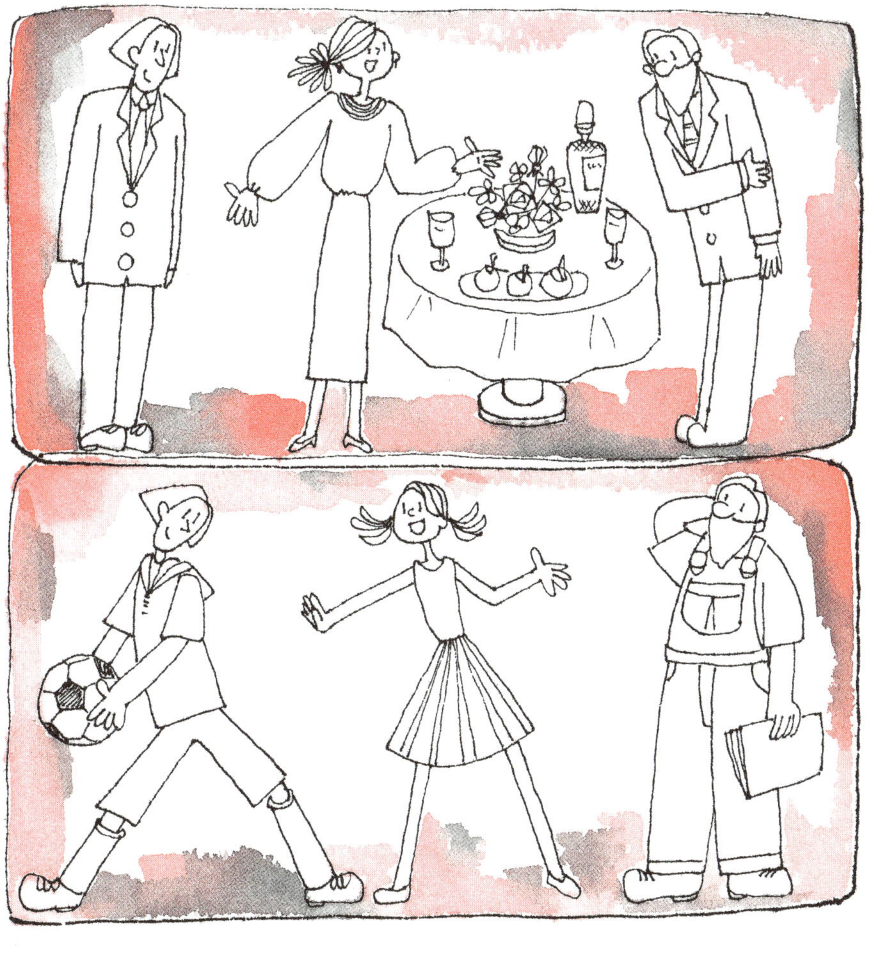

한글 번역판 참조(116P)

Activity 3: Dialog

Listen to the dialog and fill in the missing words.

CD

■ Hyoja's First Day

Head Nurse: I want to 1) ______________ you to some of the people you'll be working with. Hyoja, this is Dr. Minjun Kim. He's the chief resident on this ward. Dr. Minjun, this is Hyoja Kim. She's going to be working on this ward.

Hyoja: 2) ______________, Dr. Minjun. I'm very pleased to meet you.

Dr. Minjun: I'm glad to meet you, too. 3) ______________ to ask me about anything you don't understand.

Hyoja: I'll appreciate your help and patience until I get use to my job.

Dr. Minjun: Well, I must continue my 4) ______________ and see my patients.

Head Nurse: We have 4 nurse's aides working here and there are 15 nurses and 6 doctors assigned to this ward. There's also a receptionist who does clerical work. I'll introduce you later. Let me bring you to the 5) ______________ and you can meet the nurses who are coming off this shift.

■ In the Nurses' Lounge

Head Nurse: 6) ______________ Hyoja Kim. She's going to be your colleague. I have some work to do, so please introduce yourselves to Hyoja.

Hyoja: I'm Hyoja Kim and I'm going to be working on this 7) ______________. I'm very happy to meet you all. I know I'll have a lot of questions at first, so I hope you can show me the ropes.

Eli: Hyoja, I'm Eli Jung, and these are Jihye Kim, Inhye Kim, Dohyun Lee, and Dohee Jung. Of couse we'll 8) ______________. Please ask about anything you like.

Hyoja: Thank you. I'm really glad to meet everyone. I know I'll enjoy working with all of you.

한글 번역판 참조(117P)

Dohee: We're glad to meet our new colleague.

Eli: Where 9) ______________, Hyoja?

Hyoja: I'm from Wando. I've been working at a Red Cross Hospital in Wando for 8years. But I went to 10) ______________ in Seoul and want to live here again. Where are you from, Eli?

Eli: Oh, I'm a native of Seoul. Which nursing school did you attend?

Hyoja: I went to the nursing school attached to the National Medical Center.

Eli: Oh, me too! I graduated 5 years ago so 11) ______________. Where do you live?

Hyoja: I found an apartment 12) ______________. How about you?

Eli: I live with my parents and younger brother in Jongno. What are your 13) ______________?

Hyoja: Well, I like playing tennis and singing karaoke.

Eli: I like playing tennis, too. Let's play together sometime. And we all like singing karaoke. Let's go to karaoke on our holiday.

Dohyun: How about going next Saturday after work?

Dal, Jihye, Dohee: That's a 14) ______________!

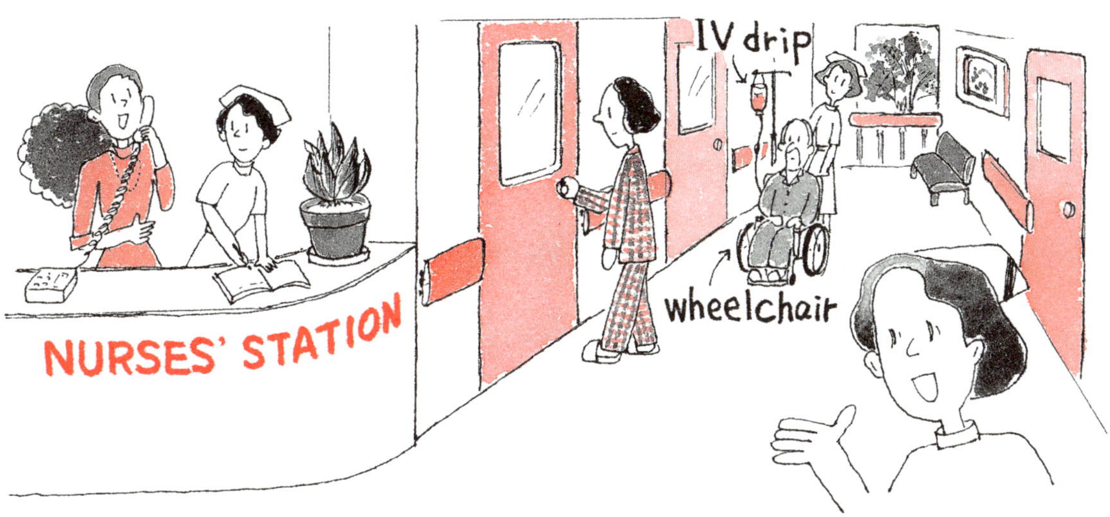

UNIT 1

Medical Terms - Departments & Occupations in a Hospital

Department of…

Internal medicine	내과
Neurology	신경과
Cardiology	순환기내과
Respiratory disease	호흡기 질환
Gastroenterology	소화기내과
Psychosomatic medicine	정신신체 의학
Pediatrics	소아과
Psychiatry	정신과
Surgery	외과
Orthopedics	정형외과
Neurosurgery	신경외과
Cardiology	심장외과
Plastic surgery	성형외과
Urology	비뇨기과
Obstetrics/Gynecology	산부인과
Dermatology	피부과
Ophthalmology	안과
Oto(rhino) laryngology, ENT	이비인후과
Dentistry	치과
Oral surgery	구강외과
Radiology	방사선과
Anesthesiology	마취과
Rehabilitation	재활의학과

Occupations

Director of nursing	간호과장
Head nurse	수간호사
Chief nurse	주임간호사
Nurse	간호사
Nurse' s aide	간호 조무사
Student nurse	간호 학생
Midwife	조산사
Doctor	의사
Resident	수련의
X-ray technician	방사선사
Lab technician	임상병리사
Dietitian	영양사
Pharmacist	약제사
Physical therapist	물리치료사
Dental hygienist	치과위생사
Receptionist	원무직원

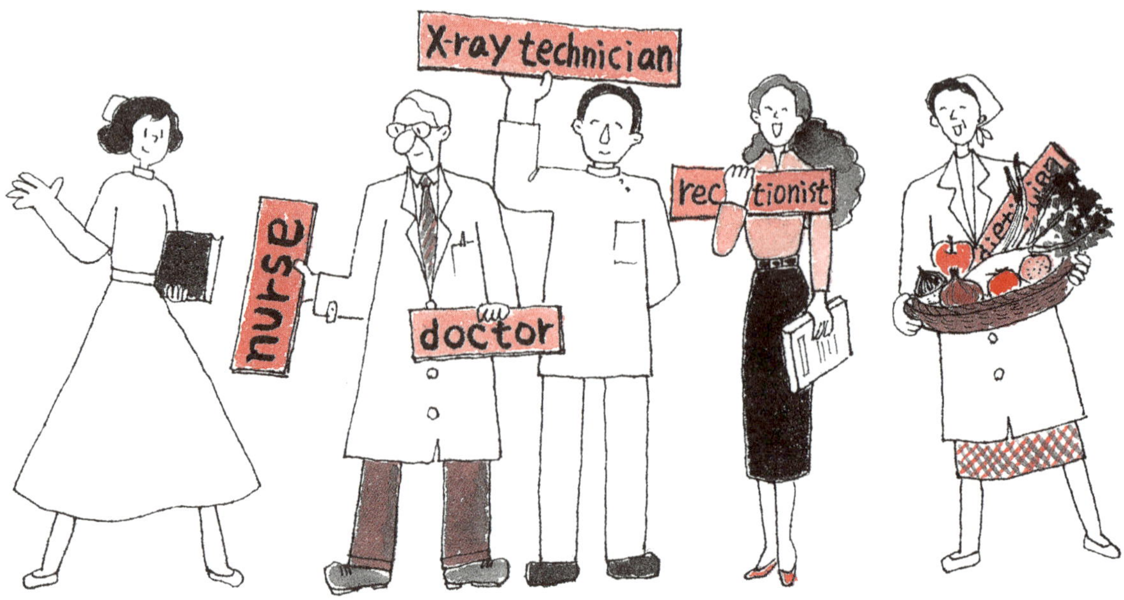

Activity 4: Puzzle-Medical Occupations-Departments

나의 직장은 어디?

다음 직종의 사람은 각각, 어느 진료과에서 근무하고 있을까요? 중앙의 문자열을 맞추어, 바른 진료과명을 우측 해답란에 쓰세요.

Job		Department
예) UROLOGIST	OYGLUOR	UROLOGY
1. MIDWIFE	ECSBTITOSR	1.
2. INTERNIST	ATNIENDECRNELIMI	2.
3. DENTAL HYGIENIST	TESINRDTY	3.
4. PEDIATRICIAN	DSEIITPACR	4.
5. X-RAY TECHNICIAN	RGOLAOIYD	5.
6. GYNECOLOGIST	EOYGYGOLNC	6.
7. CARDIOLOGIST	OCIRODALYG	7.
8. PLASTIC SURGEON	IRYTASPGUERCSL	8.
9. OPHTHALMOLOGIST	GOOLYLMPHTOAH	9.
10. PHYSICAL THERAPIST	BNAILOATIITEHR	10.
11. PSYCHIATRIST	SYYCPATHIR	11.
12. DERMATOLOGIST	OLAGREMTDYO	12.
13. ANESTHESIOLOGIST	HOLETGAOSEYSNI	13.
14. ORTHOPEDIST	IDRPHEOSTOC	14.
15. NEUROLOGIST	OYNRLEUOG	15.
16. ORAL SURGEION	ORYSAUGRLRE	16.

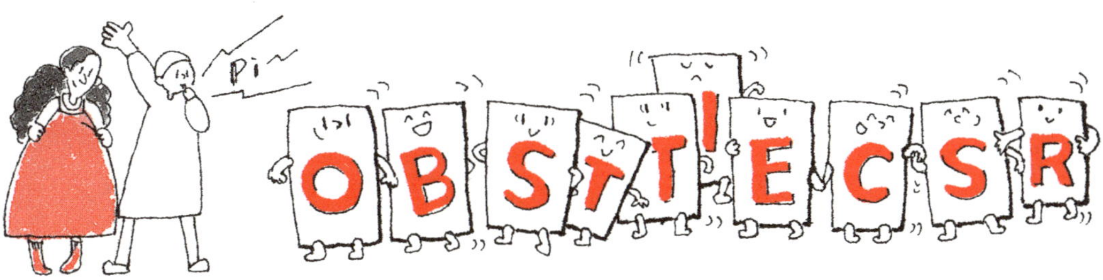

한글 번역판 참조(118P)

Activity 5: Role Play

환자의 기본정보

2인 1조가 되어, 한 사람이 간호사(A), 다른 한 사람이 환자(B) 역할을 하십시오. 아래 서류는 환자의 기본정보를 기입하기 위한 것입니다. 간호사역인 사람은 환자역인 사람에게 질문하여, 서류에 기입하세요. 끝나면 역할을 바꾸어, 환자(C)와 간호사(A)의 카드를 사용하여 연습합니다.

이 Role Play는 반드시 영어만을 사용하도록 하십시오. 상대방이 말하고 있는 것을 알아듣지 못하거나, 철자 등을 모르는 경우에는 Checkpoint에 있는 Emergency English를 사용하십시오.

Role Card A - Nurse

Your patient is a foreigner who can't speak Korean.

Ask the patient questions to fill out the form.

성명 ______________________ 남/여

국적 ______________ 생년월일 ______________

기혼/미혼 직종 ______________________

주소 ______________________________

전화(자택) ______________ 전화(근무처) ______________

가족구성 ______________________________

취미 ______________________________

한글 번역판 참조(118P)

Role Card B - Gerald Brown

Answer the nurse's questions, using the information below.

You are Irish. You were born in Dublin, Ireland on October 20, 1978. You are living with your girlfriend, Jenny. You are a dancer and a bartender. Your address is: 522-11 Sungnae-dong Kangdongku Seoul, 185-435. Your telephone number at home is: 02-6407-4328 and at work is: 02-741-4494. Your hobbies are jogging and playing soccer.

Role Card C-Patient; Mary Lee Smith

Answer the nurse's questions, using the information below

You are American. You were born in Trenton, New Jersey, in the United States on August 13, 1962. You are married and have 3 children, 10-year-old twin sons and a 12-year-old daughter. You are a dental hygienist. Your address is: Grace Mansion #407, 112-1 Inui-dong, Jongno-ku Seoul 110-717, Your telephone number at home is: 02-561-7804 and at work is: 02-471-4218. Your hobbies are reading and knitting.

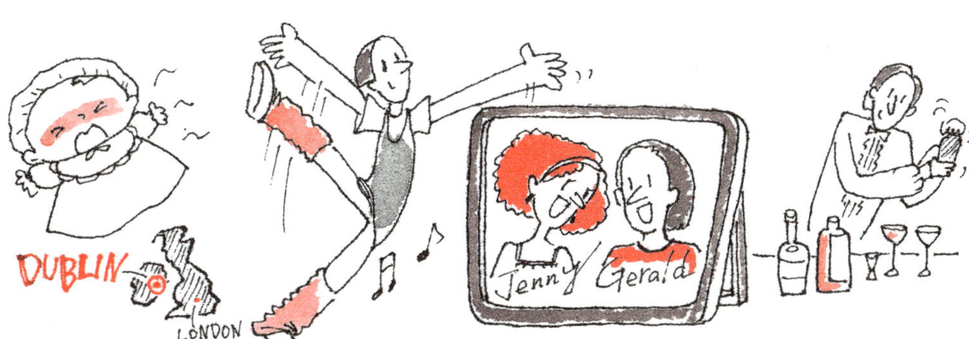

Activity 6: Game-Name Game

어디까지 기억할 수 있는가?

이 게임에서 모두의 이름과 취미를 기억합시다. 10~15명씩 그룹을 나누어 원을 만들어 주십시오. 처음 사람이 자신의 이름과 취미를 영어로 이야기합니다. 다음 사람은 자기보다 앞 사람의 이름과 취미를 모두 반복한 후에, 마지막에 자신의 이름과 취미를 말해 주십시오.

A: My name is Elie and my hobby is playing tennis.

B: Her name is Elie and her hobby is playing tennis.
My name is June and my hobby is riding a motorbike.

C: Her name is Elie and her hobby is playing tennis.
His name is June and his hobby is riding a motorbike.
My name is Sara and my hobby is social dancing.

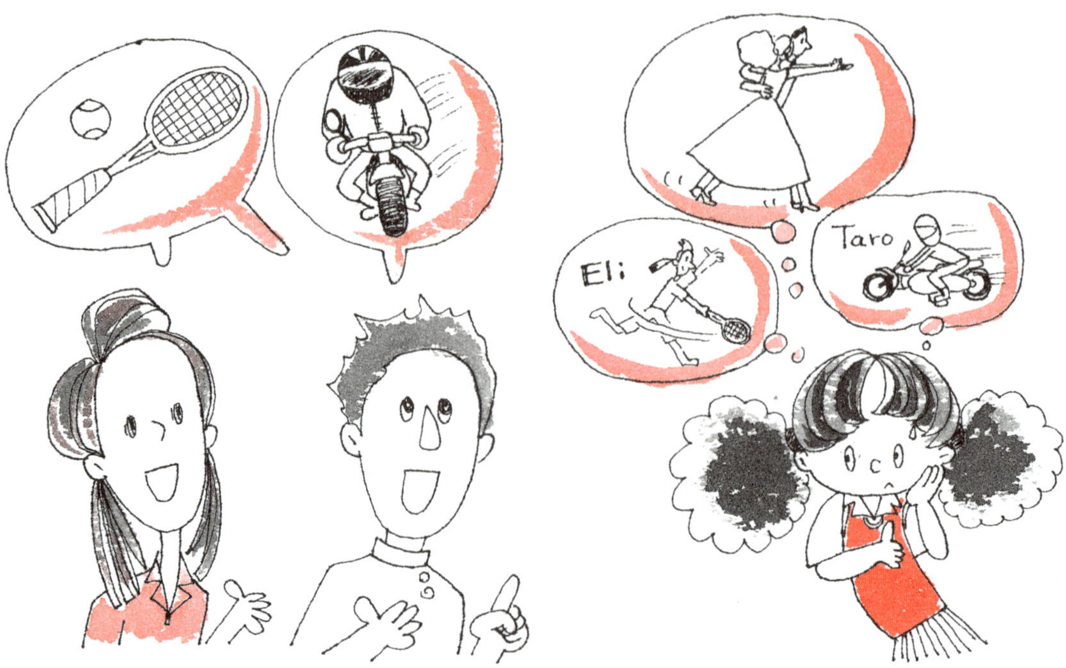

UNIT 2

What seems to be the problem today?

한글 번역판 참조(119P)

Activity 1: Listening Practice

CD 5

Listen to the conversations and choose the correct answers.

1. What is wrong with the patient?
   a) He doesn't have an insurance card.
   b) He's got lower back pain.
   c) He wants to go to the orthopedics department.

2. What are Mrs. Jefferson's symptoms?
   a) She has constipation, a cough and a fever.
   b) She has a fever, diarrhea and a cough.
   c) She has diarrhea, lower back pain and a toothache.

3. Which department should the patient go to?
   a) Plastic surgery b) Surgery c) Oral surgery

4. How long has Mr. Jones been having stomach pain?
   a) For one week. b) For two days. C) For two months.

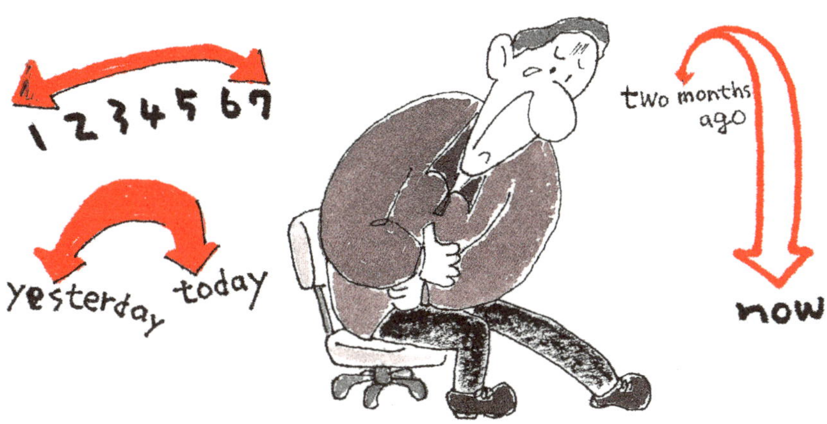

Activity 2: Checkpoint

CD 6

진료수속을 할 때

1. 이전에 병원에 오신 적이 있으십니까?
Have you visited this hospital before?
Have you been a patient here before?

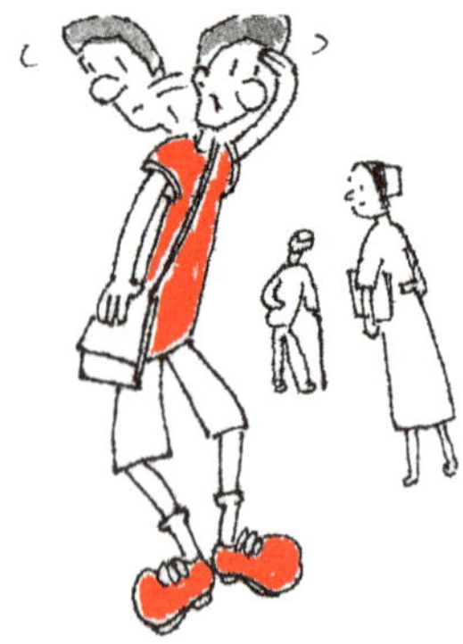

2. 이 병원 카드(의료보험 카드)를 가지고 계십니까?
Do you have this hospital's ID card(an insurance card)?

3. 무슨 과 진료를 보기 원하십니까?
What department do you want to visit?

4. 이 서류를 작성해 주세요
Please fill out(in) this form.

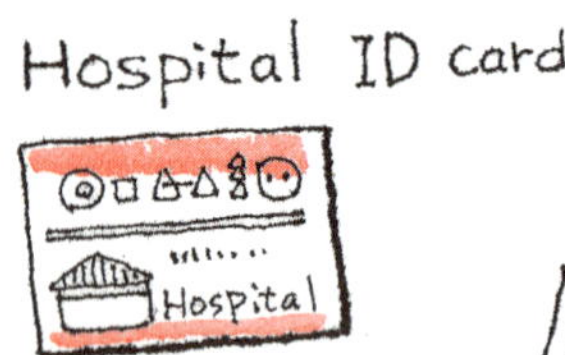

5. 키(몸무게, 나이)가 얼마 되시는지 말씀해 주시겠습니까?
Would you mind telling me your height(weight, age)?
What is your height(weight, age)?

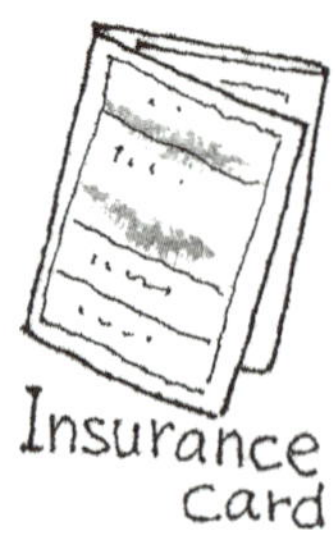

나이가 어떻게 되십니까?
How old are you?

키가 얼마 입니까?
How tall are you?

몸무게 얼마 입니까?
How much do you weigh?

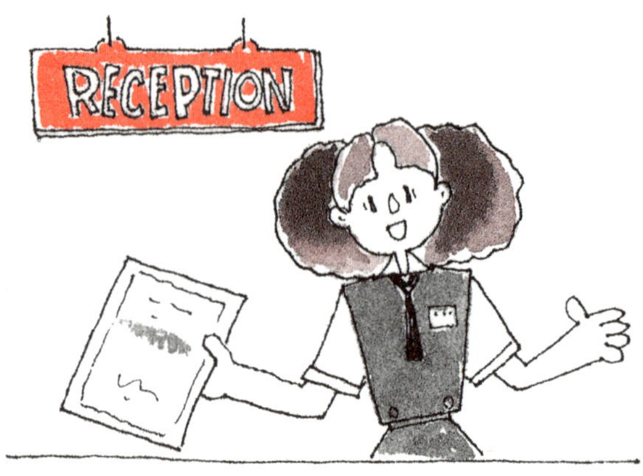

증상을 물을 때

1. 어디가 아프십니까?
What seems to be the problem?
What's the matter?

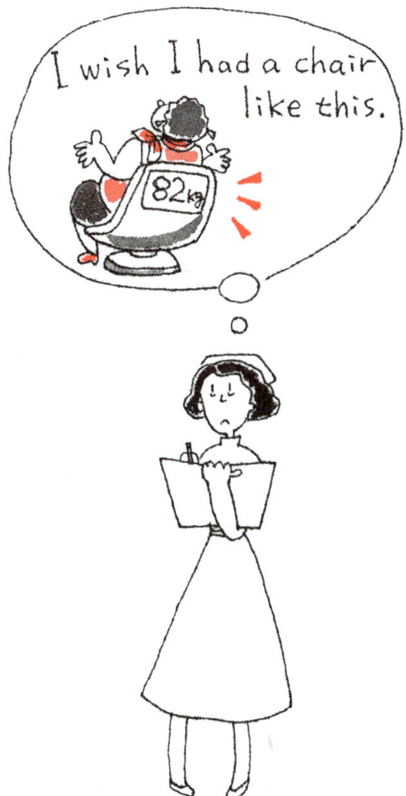

2. 어떻게 지내셨습니까?
How have you been feeling?

3. 증상은 어떻습니까?
What are your symptoms?

4. 이러한 증상은 얼마 동안 있었습니까?
How long have you had these symptoms?
How long has this been going on?

　3일(주, 달) 동안
　For 3 *days(weeks, months).*
　월요일(지난주, 지난달) 부터
　Since *Monday(last week, last month).*

5. 얼마 동안 구토(기침)를 하셨습니까?
How long have you been vomiting(had a cough)?

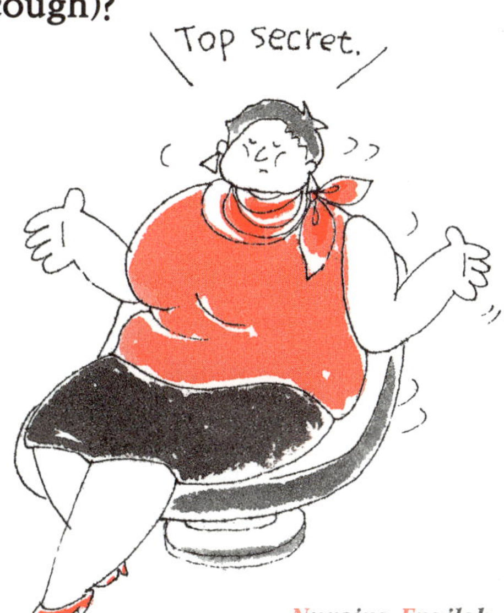

6. 설사를 몇 번 하셨습니까?
How many times did you have diarrhea?

7. 열이 납니까?
Do you have a fever(temperature)?

8. 체온이 얼마 입니까?
What's your temperature?

한글 번역판 참조(119P)

• Measurement: 측정 단위와 약어

신장

Ft = foot, feet: 피트	1ft = 12in
In = inch: 인치	1in = 2.54cm
Cm = centimeter: 센티미터	1cm = 0.394in

체중

lb = pound: 파운드	1lb = 0.454kg
Kg = kilogram: 킬로그램	1kg = 2.2lb

• Temperature 체온

°F = Fahrenheit: 화씨

°C = Celsius: 섭씨

°F = 9/5°C+32

°C = 5/9(°F−32)

Normal Body Temperature: 정상 체온

98.6°F(설하, 직장)

36.5°C(액와)

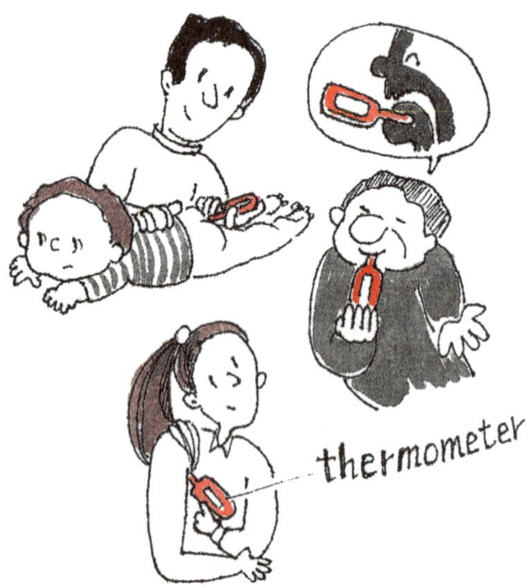

Note In korea, temperature is taken by placing the thermometer in the armpit, while in western countries, usually adults place the thermometer under the tongue and with babies or young children, the thermometer is inserted into the anus. Recently, however, a faster thermometer, one placed in the ear and measuring the temperature from the eardrum, is being used. This difference results in a slightly different figure for "normal body temperature". Only America uses pounds, feet, inches: Canada, the U.K. and Australia all use the same system of measurement as Korea.

한글 번역판 참조(120P)

Activity 3: Dialog

CD 7

Listen to the dialog and fill in the missing words.

■ In the Outpatient Clinic

Hyoja: Mr. Bergeron? Mr. Alexander Bergeron?
Mr. Bergeron: Yes?
Hyoja: 1) ______________ this hospital before?
Mr. Bergeron: Yes, I have. I was a patient here about 2 years ago.
Hyoja: Do you have this hospital's ID card?
Mr. Bergeron: Yes, here it is.
Hyoja: Can you 2) ______________________?
Mr. Bergeron: I'm sorry, I can't read Korean.
Hyoja: OK, I'll fill it in for you. Now let me ask you some questions. 3) _______________ your first and family names please?
Mr. Bergeron: Alexander is A-L-E-X-A-N-D-E-R and Bergeron is B-E-R-G-E-R-O-N
Hyoja: Thank you. OK, would you mind telling me your 4) ____________ and weight?
Mr. Bergeron: I'm 175cm tall and I 5) _______________________ 88kg. I'm a little overweight.
Hyoja: Could you tell me your age, please?
Mr. Bergeron: 6) ______________________.
Hyoja: Now, what is 7) _______________ today?
Mr. Bergeron: I've been 8) ________________ shortness of breath and sometimes I experience a tightness in my chest and palpitations.
Hyoja: 9) _______________ has this been going on?
Mr. Bergeron: For 10) _______________ weeks now.
Hyoja: How often do you feel the tightness in your chest and palpitations?

한글 번역판 참조(121P)

Mr. Bergeron: 11) ________________, especially when I exert myself-climb up stairs or walk very quickly.

Hyoja: Are you suffering any discomfort right now?

Mr. Bergeron: No, I'm not.

Hyoja: Have you had any problems 12) ________________ before?

Mr. Bergeron: No, never.

Hyoja: Have you had any medical problems before?

Mr. Bergeron: I had my gallbladder removed 13) ________________ here before.

Hyoja: Do you have a fever?

Mr. Bergeron: I don't know.

Hyoja: OK, let me take your temperature and your blood pressure. The doctor 14) ________________ in a few minutes.

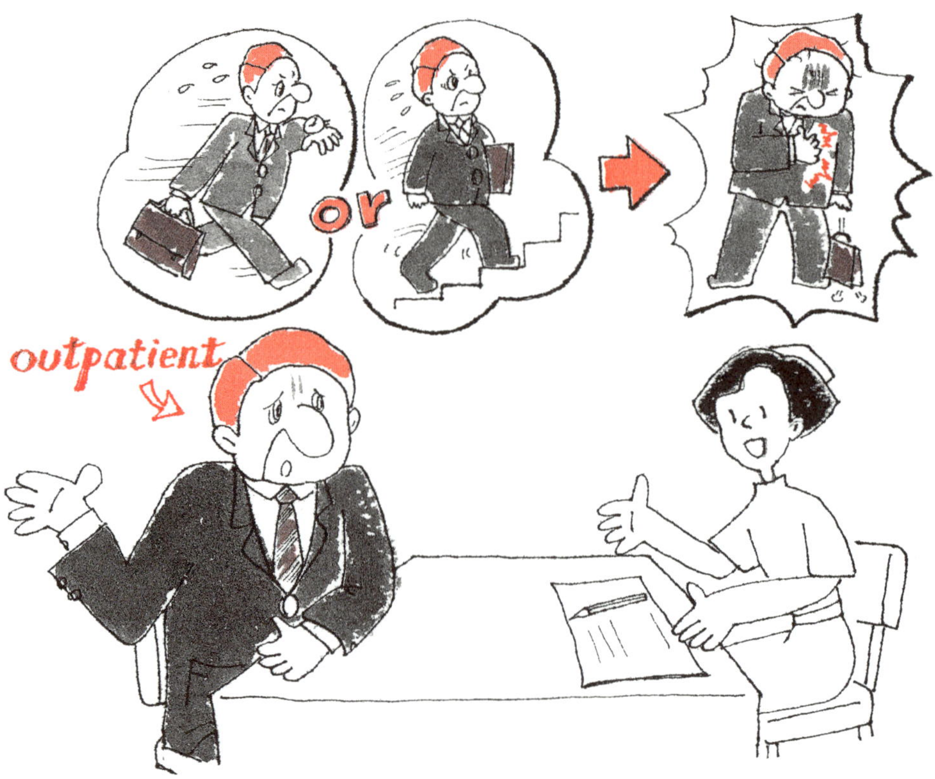

Medical Terms - Symptoms - Usage

I have…

A bloody nose	코피
bloody stool	혈변
bloody urine	혈뇨
blurred vision	흐린 시력
chills	오한
an eruption	발진
eye discharge	눈곱, 안구 이물질
a fever, a temperature	열
hiccups	딸꾹질
lesions	병변
a lump	종괴
no energy	무기력
a rash	발진
a swelling	부종, 종창

I am suffering from…

Appetite loss(gain)	식욕 부진(증가)
constipation	변비
convulsions	경련
dizziness, vertigo	어지러움, 현기증
excessive thirst	과도 갈증
hearing loss	청력 손실
heart(cold) intolerance	열(추위) 불내성
incontinence	실금, 실조
inflammation	염증
lethargy	기면
painful urination	배뇨통
weight gain(loss)	체중 증가(감소)

I have…
I am suffering from…

Abdominal pain	복통
a backache	요통
chest pain	흉통
a cough	기침
cramps	(근육)경련
diarrhea	설사
an earache	이통
gas	가스(방귀)
a headache	두통
heartburn	가슴쓰림
heart flutters	심장 떨림(조동)
insomnia	불면증
joint pain	관절통
lower back pain	요통
muscular pain	근육통
nausea	오심
pain	동통
palpitations	심계항진(가슴 두근거림)
poor digestion	소화불량
rapid heartbeat	빈맥
rectal bleeding	직장 출혈
a runny nose	콧물
shortness of breath	호흡 곤란
a sore throat	인후통
a stiff neck(shoulders)	경부(어깨)경직, 결림
a stomachache	위통
a stuffy nose	코막힘
a toothache	치통/복통, 배탈

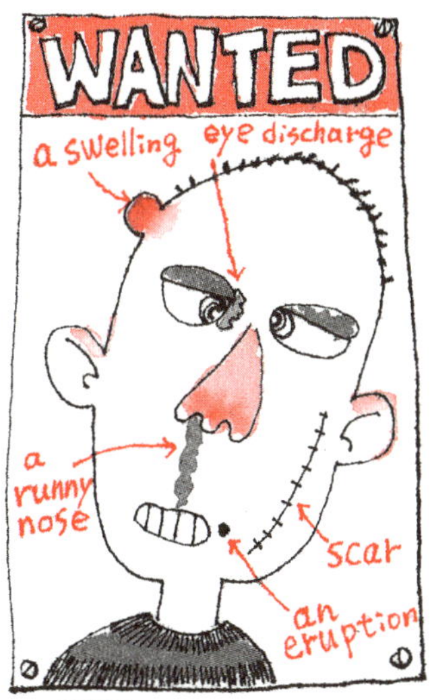

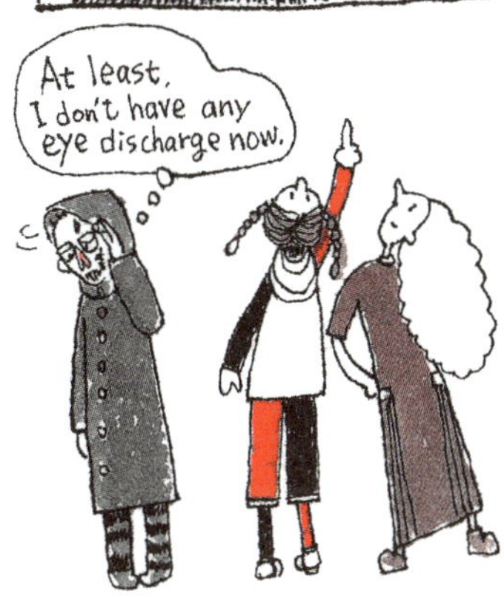

Medical Terms - Symptoms - Usage

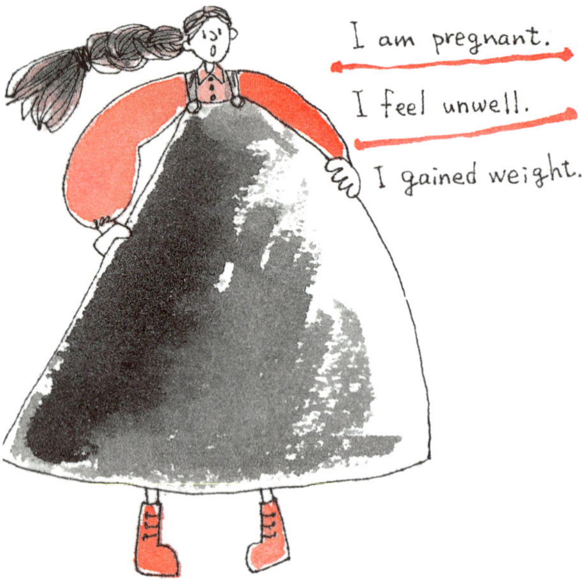

I am···

Constipated	변비인
coughing up blood	객혈이 있는
hard of hearing	듣기 어려운
having cold sweats	식은 땀이 나는
having seizures	경련이 있는
pregnant	임신 중
sneezing	재채기가 나는
sweating	땀이 나는
vomiting	구토하는
vomiting blood	피를 토한
wheezing	숨쉴 때 쌕쌕거리는

I feel···

Faint	어지러운
lethargic	졸린, 기면상태
numbness	무감각한
something stuck in my throat	목 에 뭔가가 걸린 것 같은
tightness in my chest	가슴이 조여 오는
unwell	몸이 불편한
weak	힘이 없는

I am···
I feel···

Cranky	심기가 불편한
dizzy	어지러운
gassy	가스가 찬
itchy	가려운
nauseous	매스꺼운
short of breath	숨쉬기가 힘든
sluggish	쳐지는
tired	피곤한

I···

Fainted	기절했다.
gained(lost) weight	몸무게가 늘었다(줄었다).
vomited	구토했다.
vomited blood	피를 토했다.

My···

Leg is itchy	다리가 간지럽다.
back hurts	허리가 아프다.
right(left) side is numb	오른쪽(왼쪽)이 무감각하다.
finger is swollen	손가락이 부었다.
toe is infected	발가락에 염증이 있다.

한글 번역판 참조(121P)

Activity 4: Puzzle-Scrambled Sentence

뒤죽박죽 회화

다음 회화를 바른 순서로 나열하세요. 각 문장에 번호를 붙여 주십시오.

_____ Nurse: Do you have a fever?

_____ Patient: For 3 days

_____ Nurse: What seems to be the problem today?

_____ Nurse: The doctor will see you in a few minutes.

_____ Patient: I think I have a cold.

_____ Nurse: How long have you had these symptoms?

_____ Patient: Yes, it is.

_____ Patient: I have a cough and a headache.

__1__ Nurse: Is this your first visit?

_____ Patient: Yes, I do. My temperature is 38.2°.

_____ Nurse: What are your symptoms?

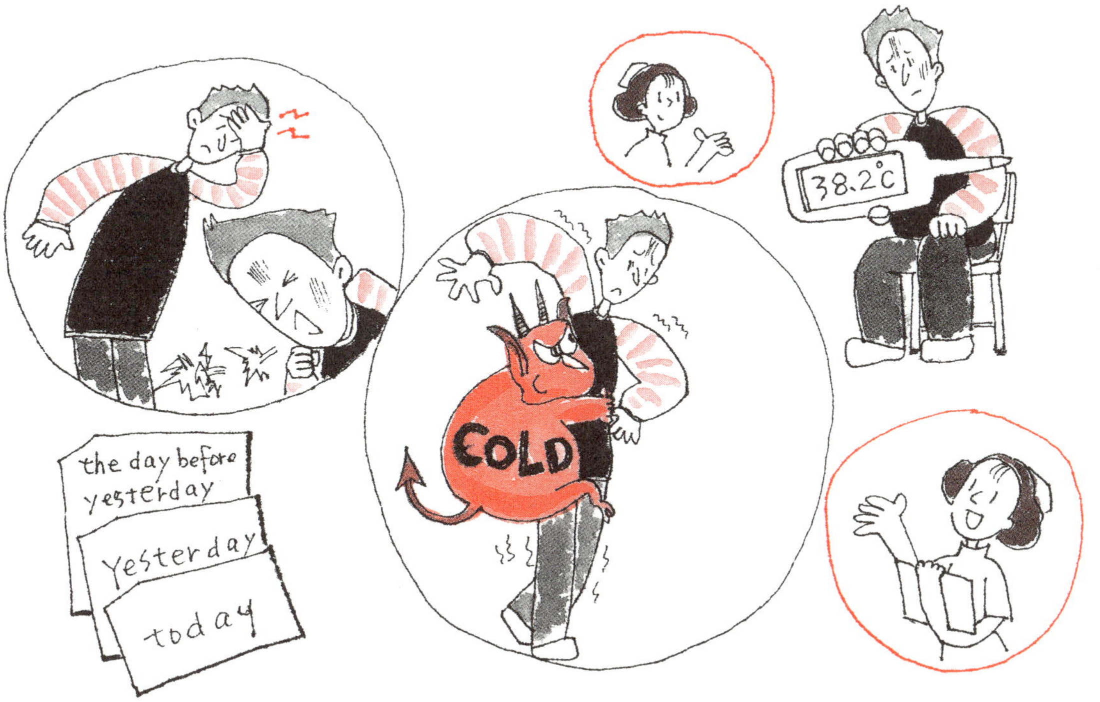

한글 번역판 참조(122P)

Activity 5: Role Play

진료신청서

2인 1조가 되어, 한사람이 간호사(A), 다른 한사람이 환자(B) 역을 합니다. 간호사는 환자에게 질문하여 서류에 기입하세요. 끝나면 역할을 교대하여, 환자(C)와 간호사(A) 카드를 사용하여 연습하십시오.

Role Card A - Nurse

Your patient is a foreigner who can't speak Korean.
Ask the patient questions to fill in the form.

진료신청서

진료과:

내과 외과 산부인과 정형외과 이비인후과 안과 재활의학과 소아과

성명 ______________________ 성별: 남/여

체중 ____________ 신장 ____________ 연령 ____________

무슨 일이 있었습니까?

어떤 증상입니까?

언제부터입니까?

몇 회 정도입니까?

한글 번역판 참조(122P)

Role Card B - Patient; Alan Moss, 29-year-old male

You weigh 155 pounds and you are 5 feet 11 inches tall. You twisted youre ankle when you were playing beach volleyball yesterday afternoon. Your ankle is very painful and swollen. You want to go to the orthopedic department.

Role Card C - Patient; Sandra Philips, 52-yesr-old female

You weigh 138 lbs and are 5 ft 6 in tall. You have pain in your right abdominal area. You have had pain and been nauseous for 3 days. Yesterday, you vomited twice. You have a fever; your temperature is 100° F. You're not sure which department you should go to. Ask the nurse.

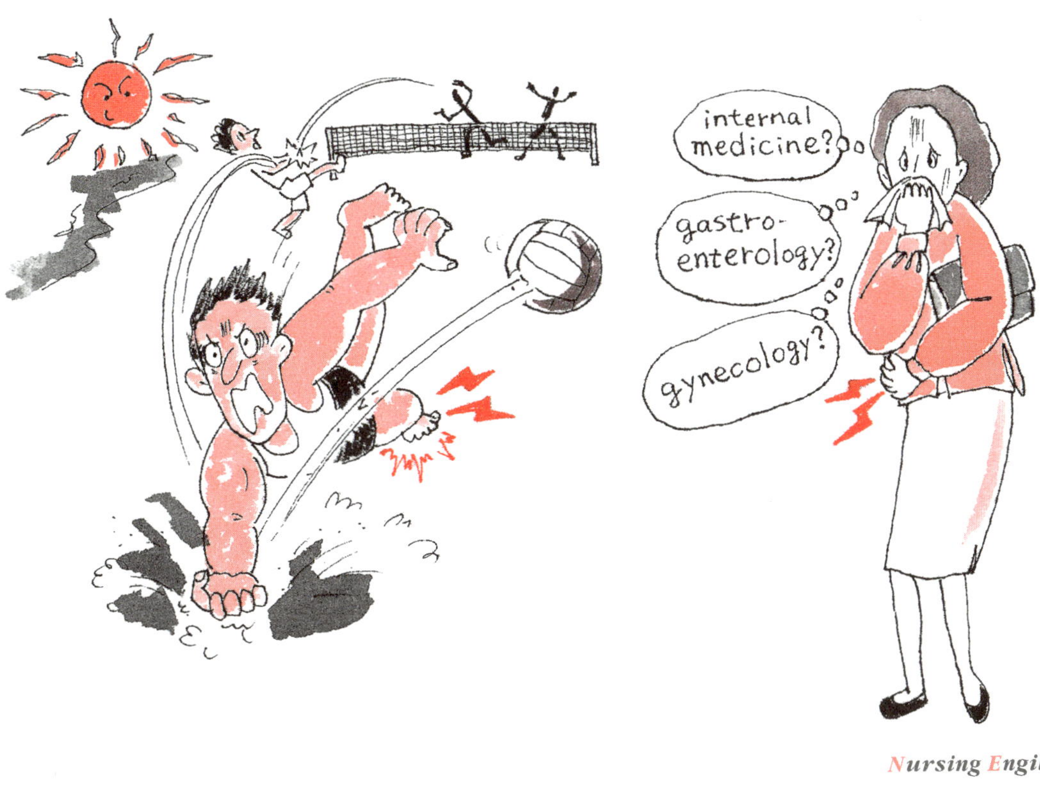

Activity 6: Game-What's the sentence?

무슨 일이 있었습니까?

이 게임은 4인 1조로 합니다. 선생님이 여러 가지 증상이 적힌 카드를 건네줍니다. 카드를 잘 섞은 다음 포개어, 책상 위에 엎어 놓으십시오. 우선 누구부터 시작할 것인가를 정하고, 다음에는 시계방향으로 합니다. 처음 하는 사람은 제일 위의 카드를 잡고, 거기에 적혀 있는 증상을 나타내는 말을 읽어 주십시오. 그러면 그 옆 사람이 그것을 문장으로 말합니다. 예를 들면 "nausea"인 경우, "I feel nauseous." "I am nauseous." "I am suffering from nausea." 처럼 대답합니다.

Nausea 메스꺼움	예) "I feel nauseous." "I am nauseous." "I am suffering form nausea."	나는 속이 메스껍습니다.

바른 문장을 말하면 카드를 받을 수 있습니다. 그 사람이 말하지 못하면 다른 사람이 대답할 수 있습니다. 카드는 바르게 말한 사람의 것이 됩니다. 아무도 대답하지 못한 경우에는 읽은 사람이 카드에 적혀 있는 답을 가르쳐 주고, 그 카드는 책상 위에 포개 있는 카드 속에 다시 한번 섞어 주십시오. 끝났을 때에 가장 많은 카드를 가지고 있는 사람이 이깁니다.

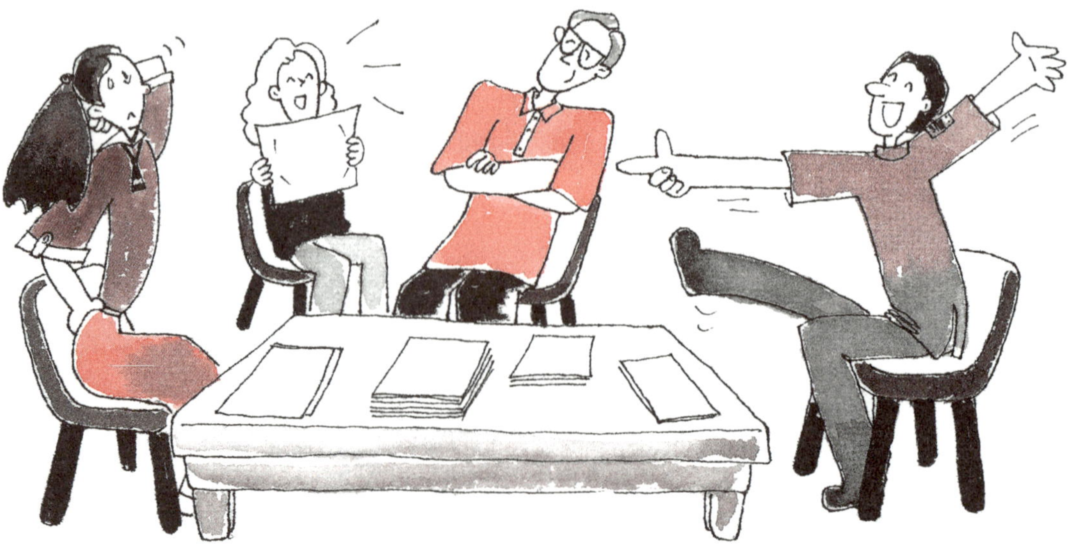

UNIT 3

This is the nurses' station.

한글 번역판 참조(123P)

Activity 1: Listening Practice

CD 8

Listen to the conversation and choose the correct answers.

1. What time are visiting hours on Sunday?
   a) from 2 to 7 pm   b) from 12 o' clock   c) from 11 to 7

2. On which days can women use the bath?
   a) Saturday, Sunday, Monday
   b) Monday, Wednesday, Friday
   c) Tuesday, Thursday, Saturday

3. Where should patients who can walk eat their meals?
   a) restaurant   b) their own room   c) dining room

4. What are the 3 places where we can find a nurse call button?
   a) dining room, patient's bed, nurses' station
   b) bath, nurses' station, toilet
   c) toilet, bath, patient's bed

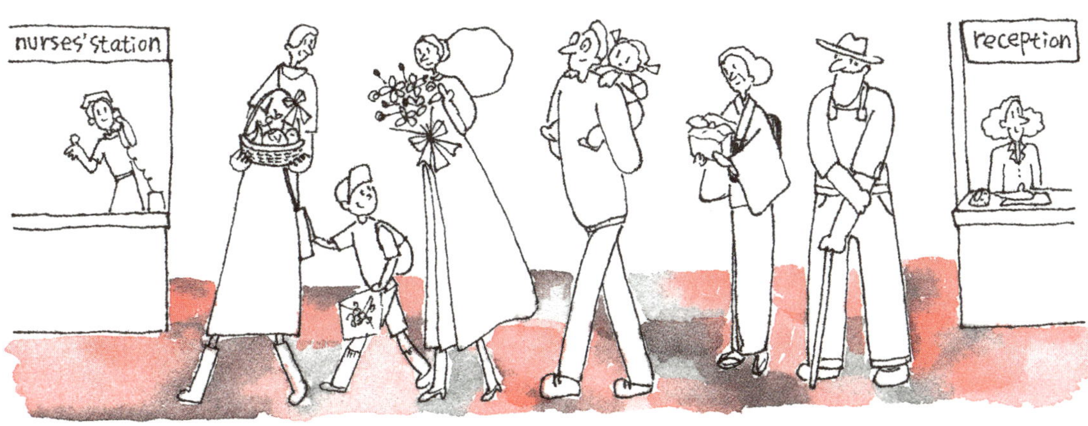

Activity 2: Checkpoint

CD 9

장소나 비품 설명하기

1. 이것이 간호사 호출 버튼입니다(식당).
This is the nurse call button(dining room).

2. 여기가 간호사실 입니다(화장실, 욕실, 샴푸실, 상담실).
Here is the nurses' station(toilet, bath, shampoo room, consultation room).

3. 여기에 공중전화가 있습니다(엘리베이터).
Here are the public telephones(elevators).

4. 욕실은 샴푸실 건너편에 있습니다.
The bath is across from the shampoo room.

5. 간호사실은 검사실 옆에 있습니다.
The nurses' station is next to the examination room.

6. 상담실은 왼쪽에 있습니다.
The consultation room is on the left(right) side.

7. 이 홀(복도)을 쭉 따라가다 왼쪽(오른쪽)에 있습니다.
It's straight down the hall(corridor) and on the left(right).

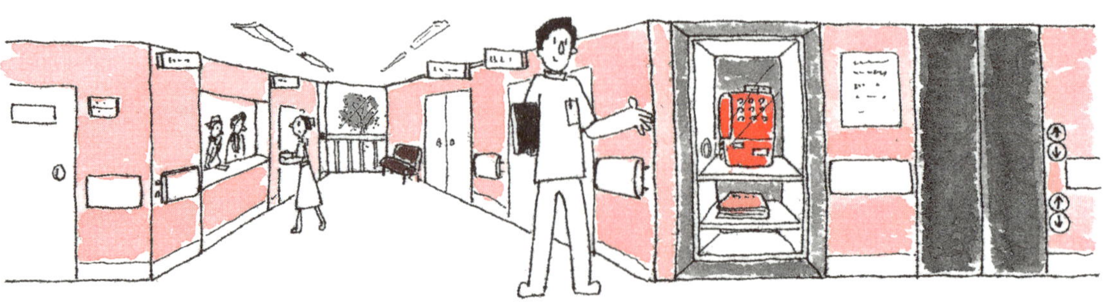

이용시간 설명하기

1. 방문객 방문 시간은 오후 2시부터 7시입니다.

Visiting hours are from 2 to 7 pm.

2. 저녁식사는 5시 30분에 제공 됩니다.

Dinner is served at 5:30

3. 오후 1시에서 4시 사이에 목욕을 할 수 있습니다.

You can take a bath(use the bath) between 1 and 4 pm.

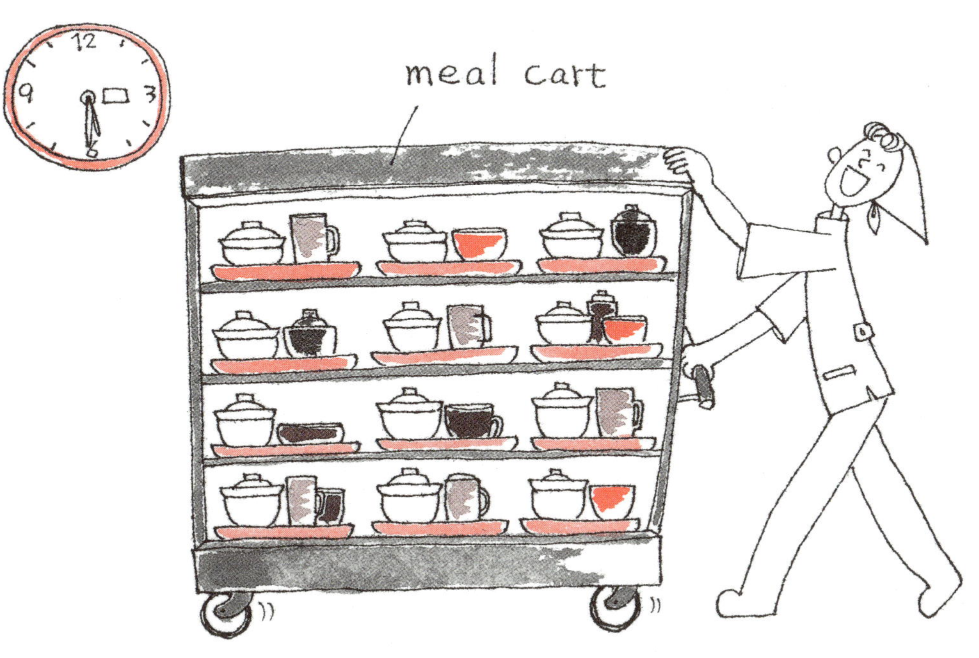

한글 번역판 참조(124P)

Activity 3: Dialog

CD 1

Listen to the dialog and fill in the missing words.

■ Admission Orientation

Hyoja: Hello Mr. Martin. I'm your 1) ____________, Hyoja Kim.

Mr. Martin: Hello.

Hyoja: Your doctor is Dr. Junsuk Park. And the 2) ____________ is Hojin Kim.

Mr. Martin: I see.

Hyoja: You can put your 3) ____________ into this locker. Put your other possessions into the 4) ____________. This is the nurse call button. Please use this if you need a nurse's assistance. Please 5) ____________ after you put away your things.

■ Later

Hyoja: Today I would like to give you an orientation 6) ____________. Please come with me.

Mr. Martin: OK.

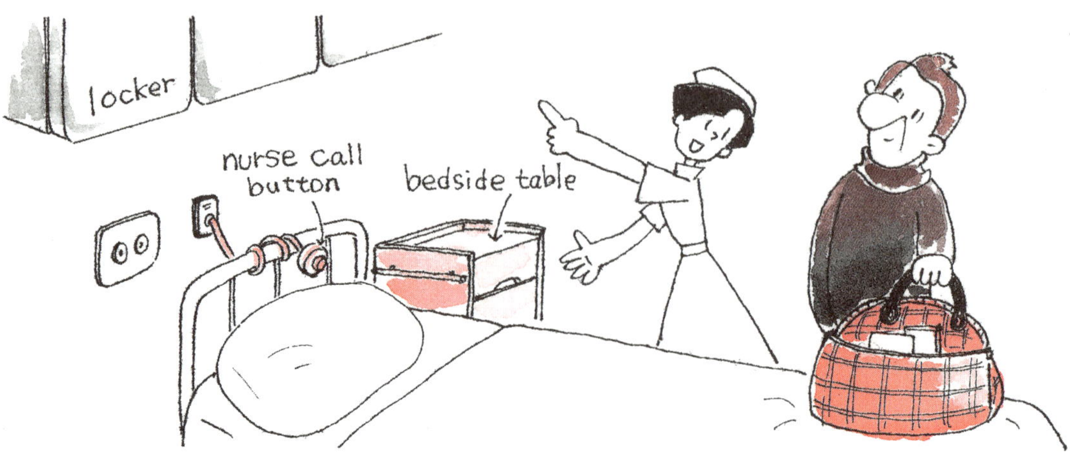

한글 번역판 참조(124P)

Hyoja: On your left is the 7) ______________. If you receive a phone call, you can get your call here. 8) ______________ the nurses' station is the consultation room.

Mr. Martin: Where can I make a phone call?

Hyoja: There are pay phones 9) ______________ outside this ward. 10) ______________ on your left. If you need to have a urine test, please put the cup in this window. On your right is the sink where you can 11) ______________ and brush your teeth.

Mr. Martin: 12) ______________?

Hyoja: You can do your laundry here. There's a coin washing machine and dryer. You can use them 13) ______________. The dining room is 14) ______________.

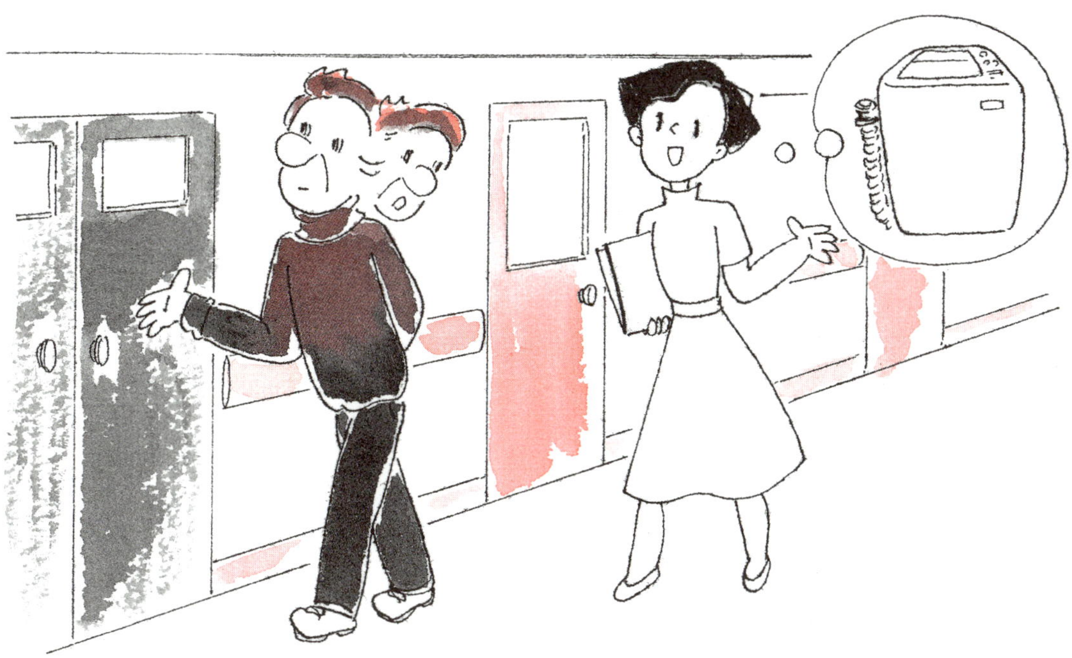

한글 번역판 참조(125P)

Activity 4: Puzzle 1-Where is it?

무슨 방이지요?

아래 힌트를 읽고 A, B, C, D, E가 각각 무슨 방인지 대답하세요.

- The dining room is across from Room 302.
- The examination room is next to the nurses' station, on the left.
- The bath is to the left of the toilets.
- The laundry is across from the nurses' station.
- The consultation room is to the right of the nurses' station.

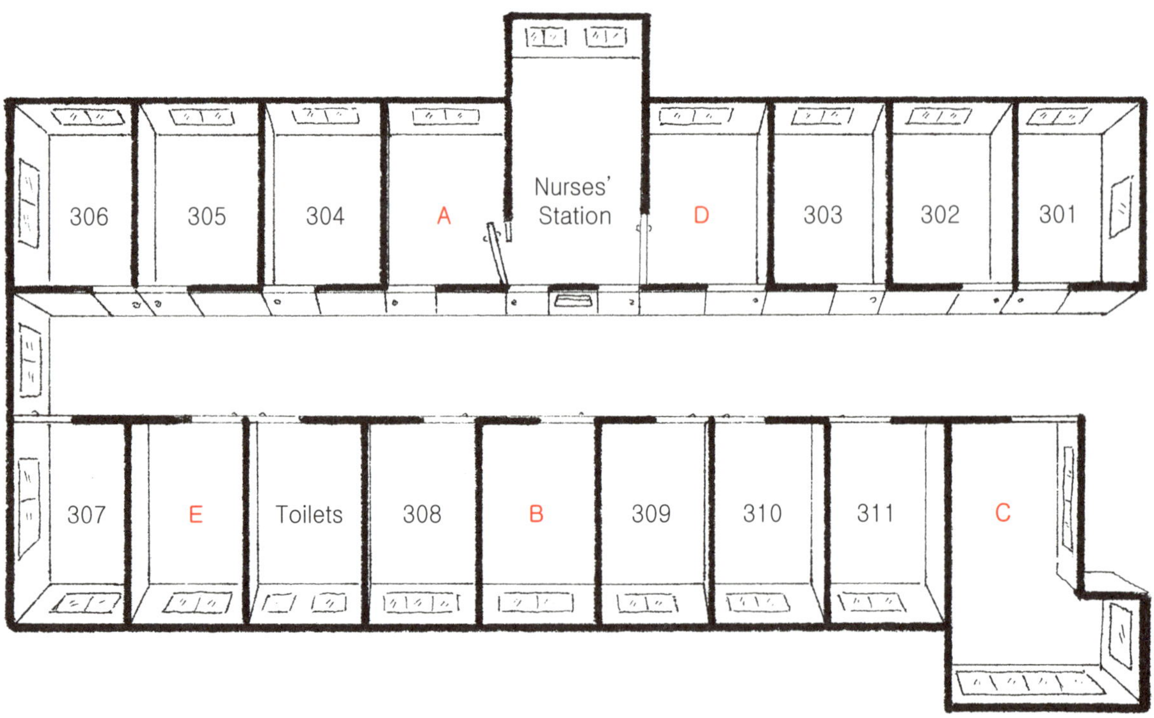

한글 번역판 참조(125P)

Activity 4: Puzzle 2-What is it?

어디에 있을까요?

병원 안에 여러 가지 비품이 있습니다. 다음 리스트에 있는 것을 그림 속에서 찾아서, 번호를 괄호 안에 쓰세요.

Objects Used in a Hospital

( ) baby bottle	( ) IV drip	( ) stethoscope
( ) bedpan	( ) latex gloves	( ) stretcher
( ) blood pressure gauge	( ) medical chart	( ) syringe(needle)
( ) case	( ) microscope	( ) thermometer
( ) crutches	( ) nurse call button	( ) vital signs monitor
( ) diaper	( ) oxygen	( ) walker
( ) emesis (kidney) basin	( ) scale	( ) X-ray
( ) examination table	( ) sling	
( ) gauze	( ) spouted water cup	

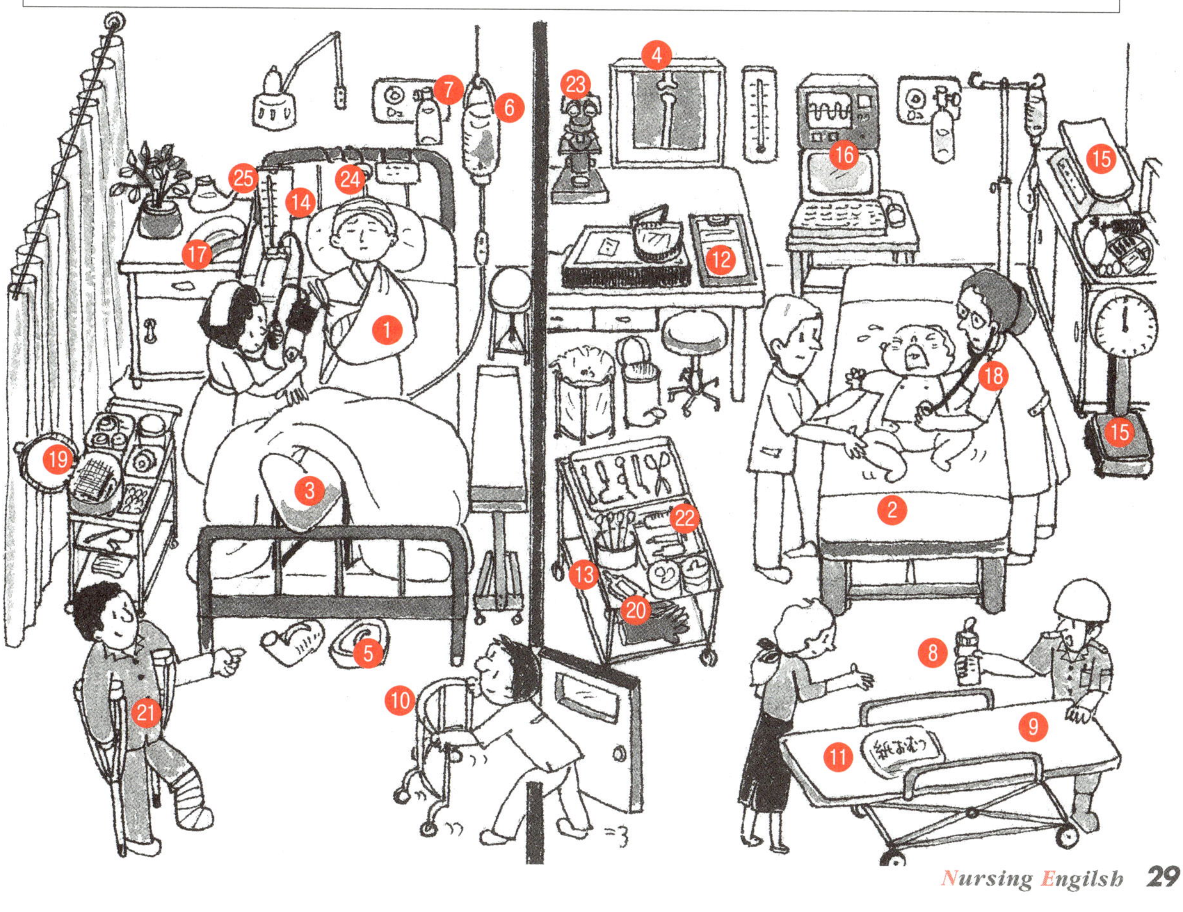

한글 번역판 참조(126P)

Activity 5: Role Play

병동안내

2인 1조가 되어 환자역(A)과 간호사역(B)을 정하고, 카드의 지시에 따라서 병동안내를 합니다. 간호사는 환자에게, 빨간글씨로 적힌 부분을 설명하십시오. 끝나면 이번에는 역할을 바꾸어, 환자(A) 간호사(C)의 카드를 사용하여 연습합니다.

Role Card A - Patient

Listen to the nurse's explanation. Ask questions. Fill in the missing information.

Your nurse: ________________ *Head Nurse:* ________________

Doctor: ________________

Visiting Hours: ________________

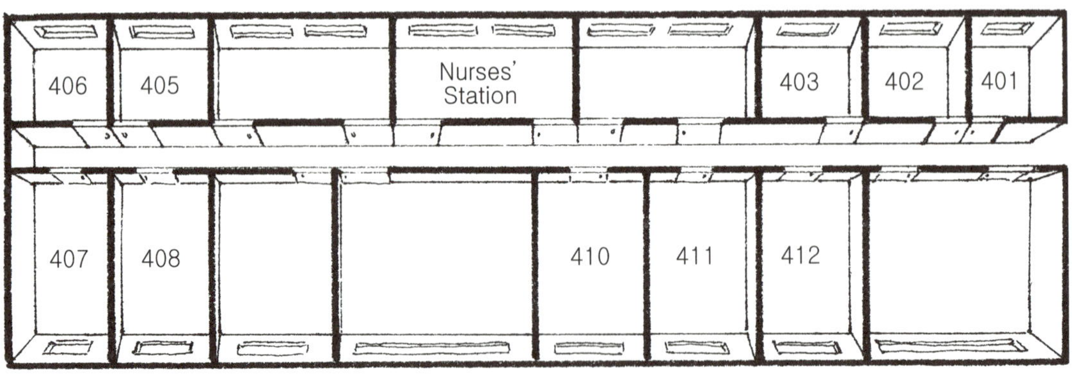

한글 번역판 참조(126P)

Role Card B - Nurse

Introduce yourself and tell the patient the information in red.

Nurse: (your name) Head Nurse: Kim Hojin

Doctor: Park Junsuk

Visiting Hours: 2 pm-7 pm

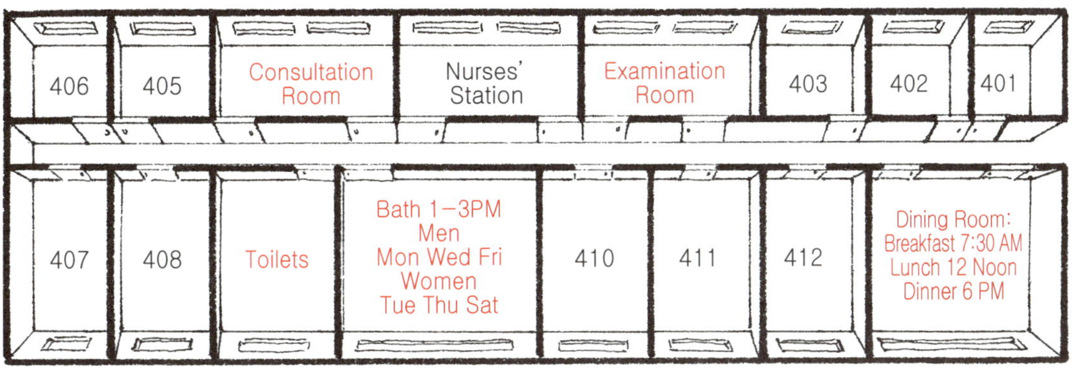

Role Card C - Nurse

Introduce yourself and tell the patient the information in red.

Nurse: (your name) Head Nurse: Kang Yoonsuk

Doctor: Kim Kyungun

Visiting Hours: 1 pm-8 pm

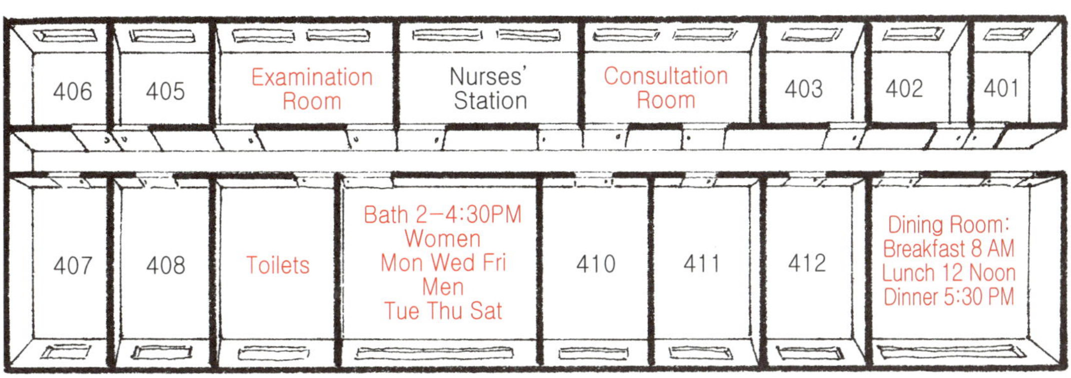

Activity 6: Game-Bingo-What time is it?

BINGO 1 카드의 눈금칸에 아래의 표에서 좋아하는 시간을 골라서 군데 군데 적어 넣습니다. 준비가 다 됐으면 빙고게임을 시작합니다. 선생님이 표 안에서 1개씩 시간을 읽어 갑니다. 당신의 빙고카드에 그것과 똑같은 시간이 적혀 있으면 그 칸을 X표시로 지웁니다. 세로·가로·대각선의 어느 쪽인가 한 줄을 전부 지우면 완성됩니다. 큰 소리로 BINGO!라고 말합니다.

8:41	2:50	5:15	10:00	11:55	6:07	1:30	12:19
6:11	12:40	4:10	7:13	9:57	1:50	11:35	2:45
12:20	6:43	9:02	12:45	7:15	2:00	5:38	3:12
7:30	1:15	3:05	3:20	5:50	6:12	2:22	4:02
8:19	10:36	7:26	11:00	12:12	4:14	5:45	1:33

BINGO 1

		FREE		

BINGO 2

		FREE		

UNIT 4 Are you suffering from any illnesses?

한글 번역판 참조(127P)

Activity 1: Listening Practice

Listen to the conversations and choose the correct answers. CD 11

1. Who is Minjun Kim?
   a) He is Ms. Cane's doctor.
   b) He is Ms. Cane's son.
   c) He is Ms.Cane's husband.

2. What restrictions does Ms. Cane have in her diet?
   a) She doesn't eat rice.
   b) She doesn't eat very salty food.
   c) She doesn't eat pork.

3. Does Ms. Cane drink alcohol?
   a) No.She quit 2 years ago.
   b) She drinks a glass every day.
   c) She drinks 7 glasses a day.

4. How did Ms. Cane's father die?
   a) He had a heart attack.
   b) He had hypertension.
   c) He had diabetes.

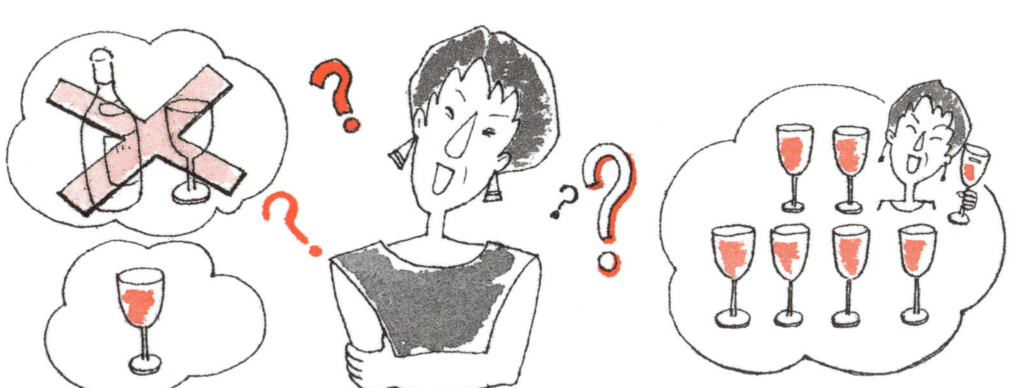

Activity 2: Checkpoint

가족력

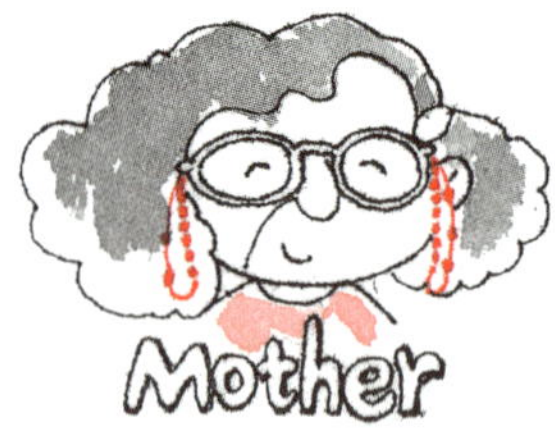

1 당신의 가까운 친지는 누구입니까?

Who is your next of kin?

2. 저희가 응급 상황 시에 누구에게 전화할 수 있습니까?

Who can we call in case of emergency?

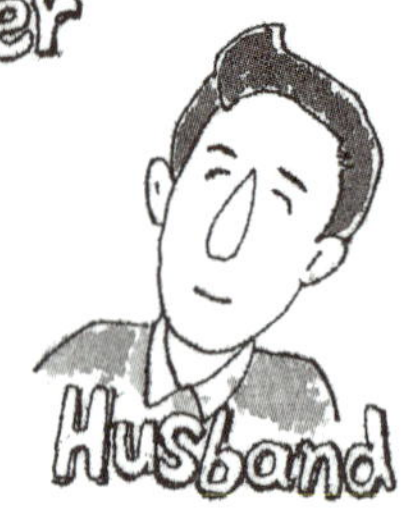

3. 당신의 가족 구성에 대해 말씀해 주십시오.

Please tell me how many people are in your family.

4. 당신의 가족 중에 병을 앓고 있는 분이 있습니까?

Does anyone in your family suffer from a disease?

　아니오/예, 어머니가 고혈압을 앓고 계십니다

　No./Yes, my mother is suffering from hypertension.

5. 그는 무엇 때문에 죽었습니까?(돌아가셨습니까?)

What did he die(pass away) from ?

　그는 간경화로 (돌아가셨습니다)죽었습니다.

　He died(passed away) from cirrhosis of the liver.

현병력 · 기왕력

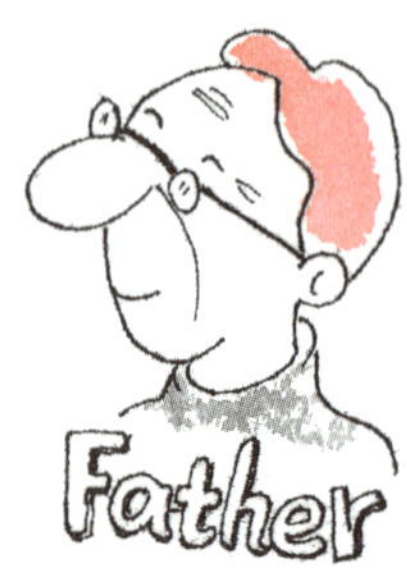

1. 당신은 앓고 있는 병이 있습니까?

Do you suffer from any illness?

　아니오, 없습니다./예, 췌장염을 앓고 있습니다.

　No, I don't./Yes, I have pancreatitis.

2. 이 병을 얼마 동안 앓고 있습니까?

How long have you had this illness?

　언제 이 병을 알게 되었습니까?

When did this illness start?

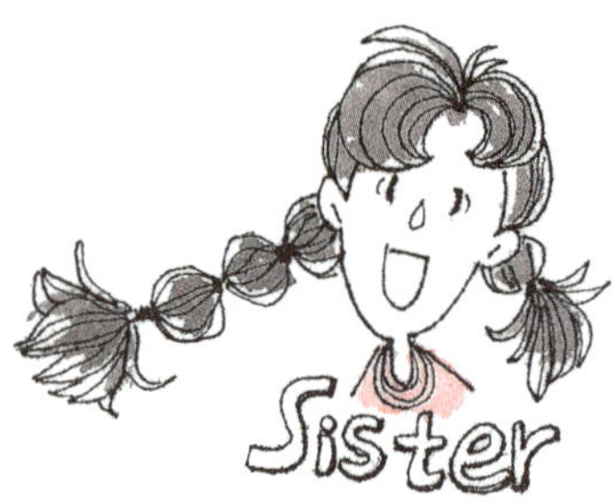

3. 당신은 심각한 질환에 걸린 적이 있습니까?

Have you ever had any serious illnesses?

　전립선암에 걸렸었습니다.

　I had prostate cancer.

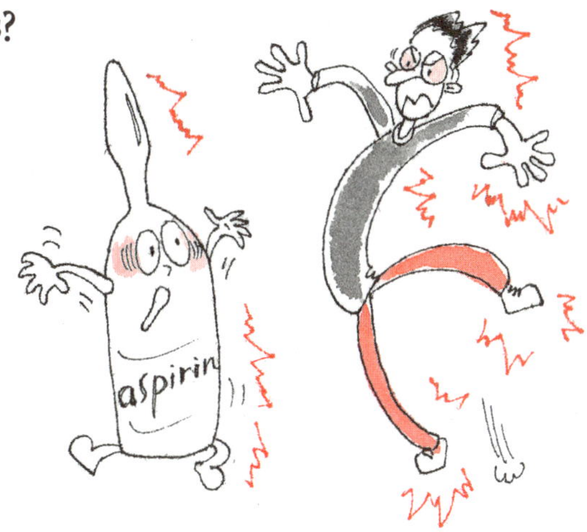

4. 그 때가 언제입니까?

When was that?

5. 당신은 알러지가 있습니까?

Do you have any allergies?

　저는 곰팡이 알러지가 있습니다.

　I'm allergic to mold.

6. 알러지가 있는 약물이 있습니까?

Are you allergic to any medication?

　예, 아스피린에 알러지가 있습니다.

　Yes, I'm allergic to aspirin.

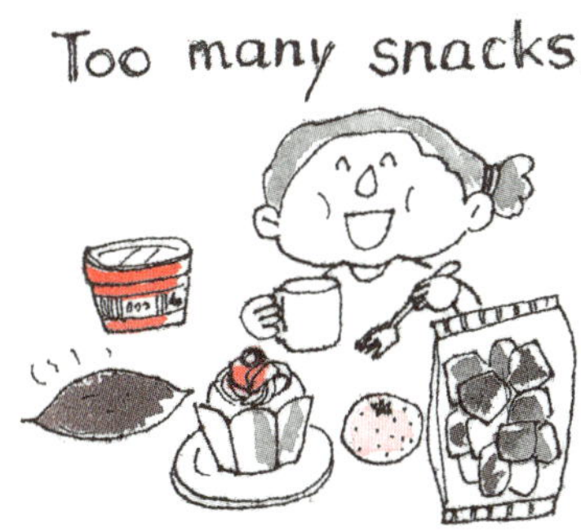

식사 · 기호

1. 당신의 일반적인 식사는 어떻습니까?

What is your usual diet?

2. 당신의 식이에 제한사항이 있습니까?

Do you have any restrictions in your diet?

　저는 돼지고기(육류, 기름진 음식, 짠 음식)을 먹지 못합니다.

　I can't eat pork(meat, fatty food, salty food).

3. 담배 피십니까(술 드십니까)? 얼마나 많이(자주) 드십니까?

Do you smoke(drink)? How much(often)?

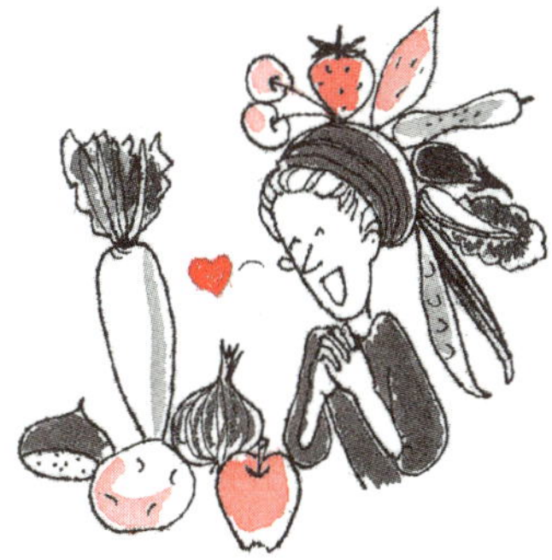

한글 번역판 참조(128P)

Activity 3: Dialog

Listen to the dialog and fill in the missing words.

CD

■ Admission Orientation

Hyoja: Is this the first time you've been admitted to a 1) __________ in Korea?

Ms. Cane: Yes, it is.

Hyoja: What is the reason for your 2) __________ today?

Ms. Cane: I have a pain in 3) __________. My doctor said it's probably appendicitis.

Hyoja: Have you ever had any serious illnesses?

Ms. Cane: I suffer from 4) __________. I also have heart disease. And I was in a car accident 3 years ago, so I can't walk.

Hyoja: Are you 5) __________ any infectious diseases?

Ms. Cane: No, I'm not.

Hyoja: 6) __________ had a blood transfusion?

Ms. Cane: No, I haven't.

Hyoja: Are you taking any medication?

Ms. Cane: Yes, 7) __________ medicine for my hypertension and heart disease.

Hyoja: Please give me your medication so I can show it to 8) __________.

Ms. Cane: OK.

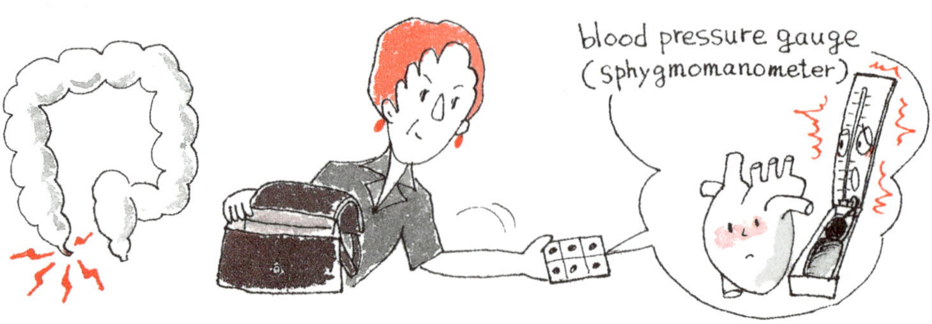

한글 번역판 참조(129P)

Hyoja: Do you have any 9) ______________?

Ms. Cane: Yes, I'm allergic to peanuts.

Hyoja: Are you allergic to any medication?

Ms. Cane: No, I'm not.

Hyoja: Do you need any help with your 10) ______________, for example with bathing or with your meals?

Ms. Cane: Well, I use a wheelchair, so I need a little help, getting in and out of the 11) ______________. But I can usually bathe myself and I do the cooking in my house.

Hyoja: How is your eyesight and hearing?

Ms. Cane: My 12) ______________ are great.

Hyoja: How would you describe your 13) ______________?

Ms. Cane: I think I'm cheerful and outgoing.

Hyoja: Could you tell me your religion?

Ms. Cane: I'm Protestant.

Hyoja: Are you concerned or 14) ______________ your illness or admission?

Ms. Cane: I'm concerned about my surgery. And I'm worried that my nurses and doctor won't be able to speak English.

Hyoja: Please, don't worry. Your doctor 15) ________________________. Some nurses can speak English, and you can ask for me if you need to talk about something.

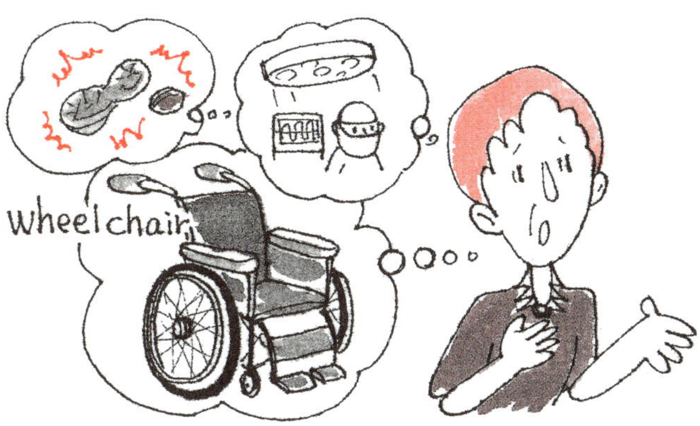

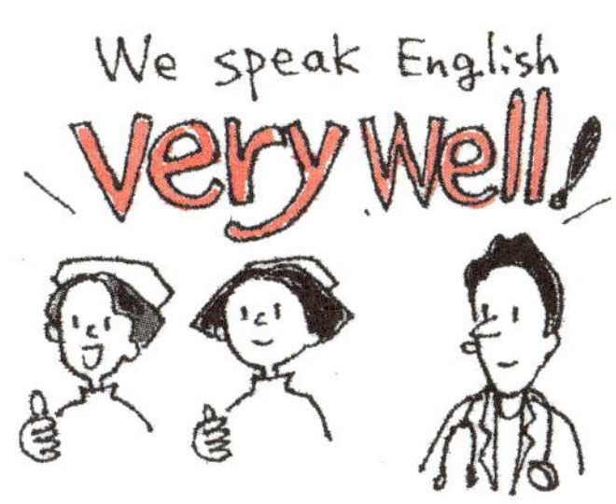

Medical Terms - Diseases & Disorders

Heart Diseases

angina pectoris	협심증
arrhythmia	부정맥
congestive heart failure	울혈성 심부전
myocardial infarction	심근경색증

Lung Diseases

(bronchial) asthma	(기관지) 천식
pleurisy (pleuritis)	늑막염
pneumonia	폐렴
pulmonary infarction	폐경색

Gastrointestinal Diseases

appendicitis	충수염
duodenal ulcer	십이지장궤양
gastric(stomach) ulcer	위궤양
gastroenteritis	위소장염
hemorrhoid(s)	치질
irritable bowel(colon)	과민성 대장

Liver, Gallbladder, Pancreas, Kidney Diseases

cirrhosis	간경화
gallstone(s)	담석
hepatitis A,B,C	간염 A, B, C
kidney stone(s)	신석증
pancreatitis	췌장염

Brain, Spinal, Nerve Diseases

Alzheimer's disease	알츠하이머 질환
cerebral hemorrhage	뇌출혈
cerebral infarction	뇌경색
epilepsy	간질
meningitis	뇌막염
migraine(headache)	(편)두통
Parkinson's disease	파킨스씨 질환
stroke	뇌졸중

Blood Diseases

anemia	빈혈
hemophilia	혈우병
leukemia	백혈병

Infectious Diseases

AIDS	에이즈
cholera	콜레라
common cold	감기
HIV	사람면역결핍바이러스
influenze(flu)	독감
malaria	말라리아
tuberculosis	결핵

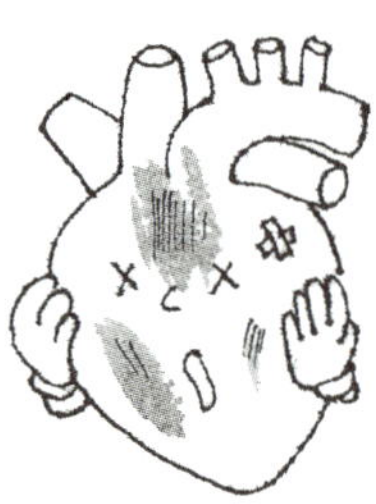

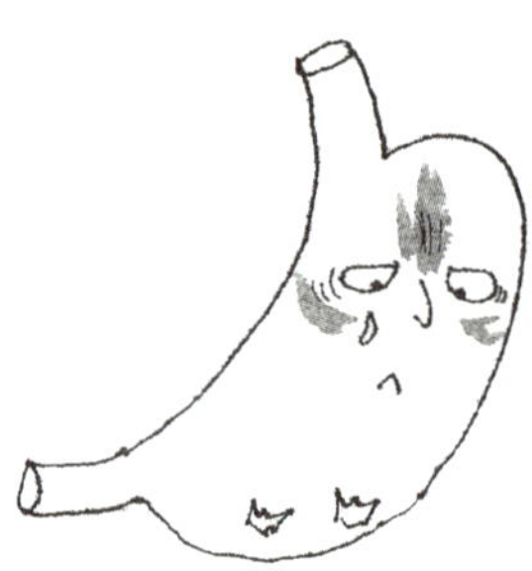

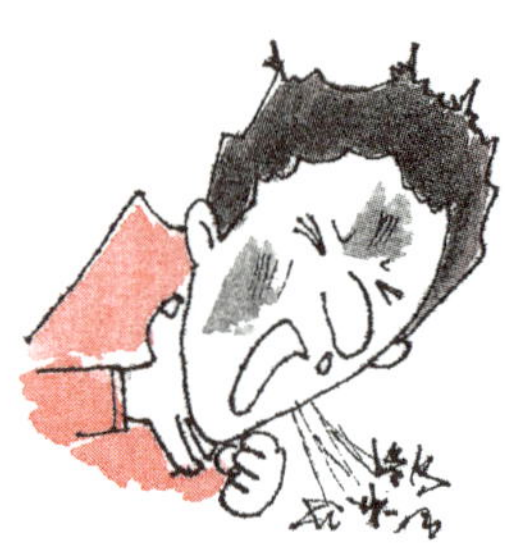

Medical Terms - Diseases & Disorders

Skin Diseases

athlete's foot	무좀
eczema	습진
hives	두드러기

Skeletal, Muscular Diseases

fracture	골절
herniated disc	추간판탈출증
osteoporosis	골다공증

Eye Diseases

cataract	백내장
glaucoma	녹내장

Ear, Nose, Throat Diseases

laryngitis	후두염
Ménière's disease	메니에르병
tonsillitis	편도선염

Other

Alcoholism	알코올중독증
allergy	알러지
anorexia(nervosa)	식욕부진(신경성)
cystitis	방광염
diabetes mellitus	당뇨병
gout	통풍
hypertension(high blood pressure)	고혈압
Hyperthyroidism	갑상선 기능 항진증
hypothyroidism	갑상선 기능 저하증
lupus(systemic lupus erythematosus)	낭창(전신성 홍반성 낭창)
Rheumatoid arthritis	류마티스 관절염

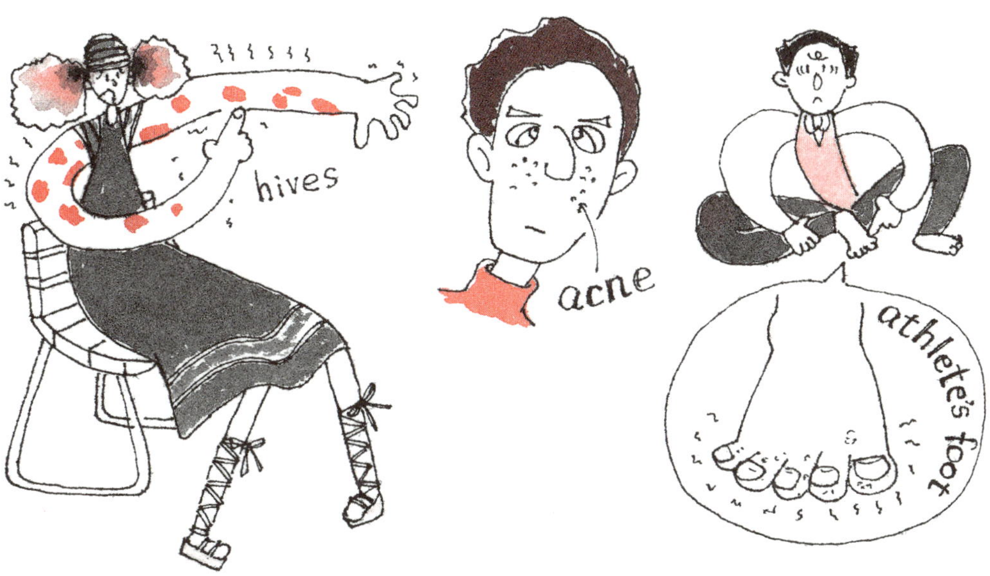

Activity 4: Puzzle-Diseases Word Search

잠복하고 있는 병은?

다음 그림의 가로·세로·대각선으로 18개의 병명이 감추어져 있습니다. 찾아내어 동그라미로 표시하세요.

U	A	A	C	A	T	A	R	A	C	T	Q	R	E	A
W	X	S	P	L	E	U	K	E	M	I	A	S	M	F
H	L	E	T	P	K	S	S	N	A	A	A	E	F	X
S	A	P	T	H	E	A	E	D	B	E	Z	D	R	E
I	S	I	B	U	M	N	H	Y	S	C	B	U	A	E
S	I	L	R	B	O	A	D	I	E	Y	X	P	C	N
O	T	E	E	V	B	G	D	I	Q	X	V	A	T	O
L	I	P	D	A	L	T	A	V	C	R	M	J	U	T
U	L	S	E	H	R	I	J	M	D	I	B	M	R	S
C	L	Y	V	A	D	P	O	L	P	S	T	L	E	L
R	I	G	E	S	C	B	M	T	L	Z	E	I	Y	L
E	S	H	D	I	A	B	E	T	E	S	P	V	S	A
B	N	H	E	P	A	T	I	T	I	S	L	U	I	G
U	O	K	M	M	S	I	L	O	H	O	C	L	A	H
T	T	L	N	O	I	S	N	E	T	R	E	P	Y	H

Challenger! 영어 병명 아래에 각각 한국어명을 적으세요. Medical Terms의 병명리스트를 보지 않고 몇 개나 할 수 있습니까?

1. ASTHMA ______
2. AIDS ______
3. ALCOHOLISM ______
4. APPENDICITIS ______
5. CATARACT ______
6. DIABETES ______
7. ECZEMA ______
8. EPILEPSY ______
9. FRACTURE ______
10. GALLSTONE ______
11. GOUT ______
12. HEART DISEASE ______
13. HEPATITIS ______
14. HIVES ______
15. HYPERTENSION ______
16. LEUKEMIA ______
17. TONSILLITIS ______
18. TUBERCULOSIS ______

한글 번역판 참조(130P)

Activity 5: Role Play

병력의 청취

2인 1조가 되어 간호사역(A)과 환자(B)를 정하십시오. 오른쪽 서류는 입원시에 환자의 병력 등을 기록하기 위한 것입니다. 간호사는 환자에게 질문하여 서류에 기입합니다. 끝나면 역할을 바꾸어 환자(C)와 간호사(A)의 카드를 사용하여 연습합니다.

Role Card A - Nurse

You are conducting an admission interview. Ask the patient about his/her family composition and family's medical history, patient's medical history, diet, dietary restrictions, smoking and drinking habits, religion and personality. Fill in the form.

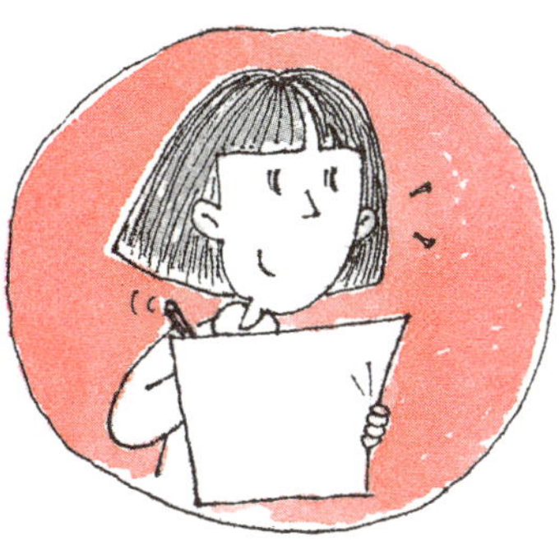

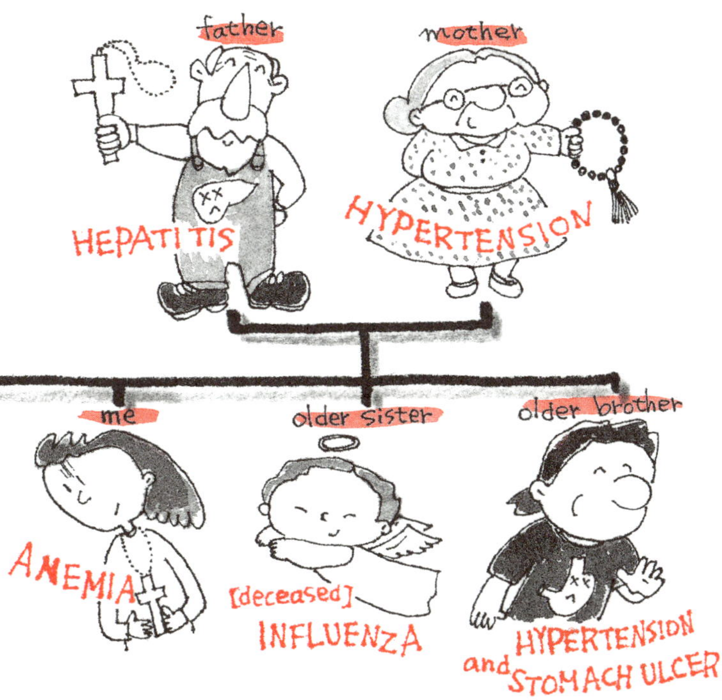

성명 ______________ 연령 ______________ 성별 ______________

1. **가족력**(가족구성, 가족병력)

2. **환자병력**

· 기왕력 발병시기 · 기간

· 현병력 발병시기 · 기간

· 알러지 유무

3. **생활력**

· 일상적인 식사

· 식사제한

· 음주 · 흡연

4. **종교**

5. **성격**

Personality

Anxious	불안한	Friendly	정다운	Shy	부끄러워하는
Calm	차분한	Nervous	신경질적인	Optimist	긍정적인
Cheerful	명랑한	Outgoing	외향적인	Pessimist	염세주의적인
Depressed	우울한	Quiet	조용한	Worrier(worrywart)	소심하고 걱정인 많은
		Serious	심각한		

한글 번역판 참조(130P)

Role Card B - Patient; Norma James, 39-year-old female

You are married. Your husband's name is Bob James. He is 43 years old. You have 2 children, an 8-year-old son, Rodney and a 12-year-old daughter, Mary. Your mother and father are alive. Your mother has been suffering from Alzheimer's disease for 2 years. Your father has been suffering from diabetes mellitus for 3 years. You have a younger brother who is healthy.

You have been suffering from asthma since you were 5 years old and had cervical cancer last year. You had a hysterectomy and are fine now. You are allergic to penicillin and peanuts.

You eat 3 meals a day. You don't eat pork and shellfish because you are Jewish. You don't smoke, but drink a glass of wine or beer almost every day.

Your personality is outgoing and cheerful.

Role Card C - Patient; Steven Anderson, 53-year-old male

You are a homosexual. You live with your partner whose name is Andrew Philips. He is 49 years old. Your mother is alive, but your father died 4 years ago from a stroke at the age of 79. He was suffering from heart disease for a long time. Your mother, who is 75, had her gallbladder removed 4 years ago. You have 2 younger sisters, Cynthia, who is 50 and Ellen, who is 48. Cynthia has gallbladder disease, but Ellen is healthy.

You have been suffering from HIV since 1997. You have had a cough for 2 months. You area allergic to dust, mold and pollen.

You are a vegetarian; you don't eat any meat or fish. You don't smoke, but drink occasionally. You are Protestant.

Your personality is serious and you are nervous and a worrywart.

Activity 6: Game-Have you ever?

~해본적 있습니까?

당신의 클라스메이트가 지금까지 어떤 경험을 했는가, 다음 질문을 5사람에게 묻고 YES/NO를 기입하세요.　예) "Have you ever been injured?"

Have you ever	Name	Name	Name	Name	Name
been	injured?	to China?	to Hawaii?	admitted to the HOSPITAL?	to the U.S.?
eaten	Mexican food?	chocolate pudding?	at a Buddhist temple?	French food?	snake?
seen	Kabuki?	Surgery?	a traffic accident?	a Namie Amuro concert?	someone fall off a bicycle?
	had stitches?	had a fever of 40℃?	had an injection?	suffered from the flu?	visited someone in the hospital?

UNIT 5

You need to have an MRI.

한글 번역판 참조(131P)

Activity 1: Listening Practice

Listen to the conversations and choose the correct answers. CD 14

1. What is the nurse doing?
   a) taking the patient's pulse   b) taking a blood sample
   c) doing a blood pressure test   d) doing an eye test

2. When should Mr. Silver have the tests done?
   a) during his surgery   b) today
   c) after his surgery   d) after his admission

3. Which part of Ms. Jackson's body does the doctor want to examine?
   a) her mouth   b) her stomach   c) her heart   d) her colon

4. What test does Mr. Kim need to have?
   a) an RI   b) an X-ray   c) an EEG   d) an MRI

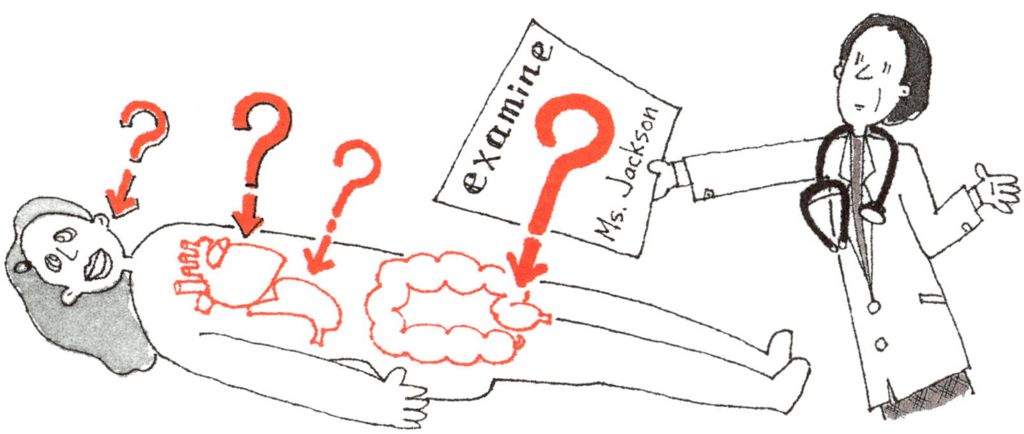

Activity 2: Checkpoint

CD 15

검사 지시를 한다.

1. 당신은 엑스레이(뇌파검사, 심초음파, 대장내시경)검사를 받아야 합니다.
You need to have an X-ray(EEG, Echogram, colonoscopy).

2. 옷을 벗으시고, 이 가운을 입으세요.
Please take off your clothing and put on this gown.

3. 이 테이블 위에 누우십시오.
Please lie on this table.

4. 오른쪽으로(얼굴을 위로하고, 얼굴을 아래로) 누우십시오.
Please lie on your right side(face up, face down).

5. 여기 서 계십시오.
Please stand here.

6. 움직이지 마세요.
Please don't move.

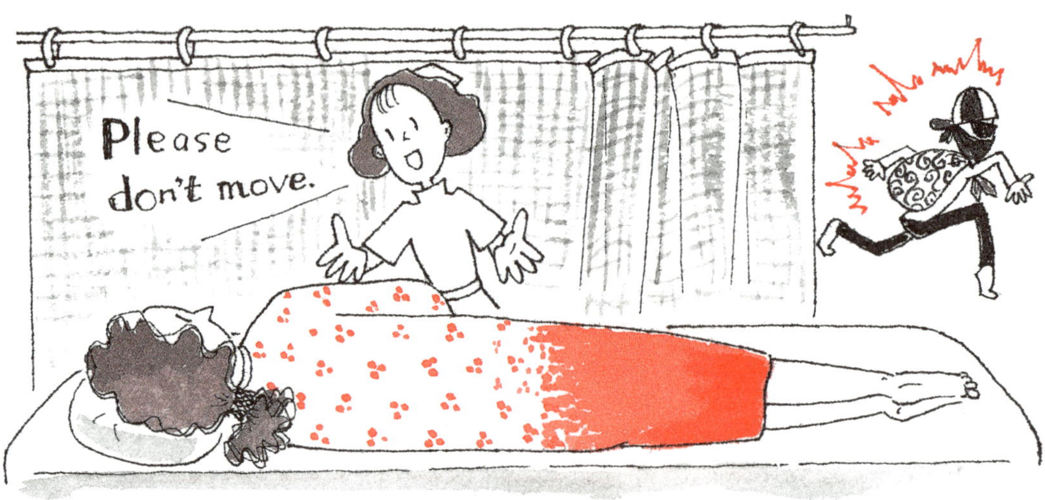

7. 주먹을 쥐세요.
Make a fist.

8. 숨 들이마시세요(내쉬세요).
Inhale(Exhale).

9. 숨을 들이마시고(내쉬고) 숨을 참으세요.
Please. Inhale(Exhale) and hold your breath.

10. 심호흡을 하세요.
Please. Take a deep breath.

11. 이 약(알약)을 드십시오.
Take this medicine(these tablets).

12. 체온을 재십시오.
Take your temperature.

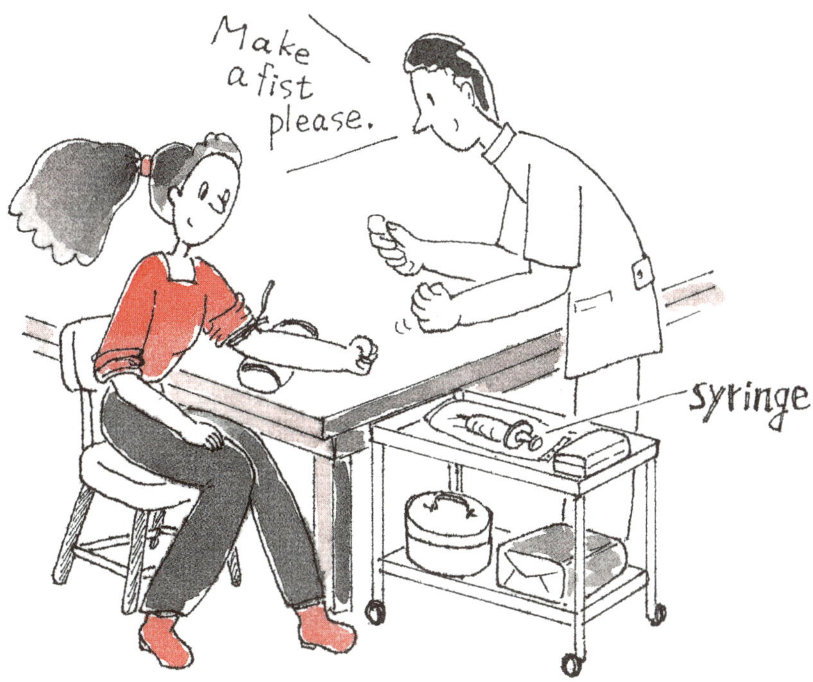

한글 번역판 참조(132P)

Activity 3: Dialog

CD

Listen to the dialog and fill in the missing words.

■ Hospital Tests

Hyoja: Ms. Smith, you need to have 1) ______________ done this week.

Ms. Smith: What tests do I need?

Hyoja: You need to have a chest 2) ______________, an EKG, a gastroscopy and an upper and lower GI series.

Ms. Smith: I've had a 3) ______________ X-ray and an EKG before, but I never had a gastroscopy or GI series before. What kinds of tests are they?

Hyoja: A gastroscopy and an upper GI series are to examine 4) ______________. In a gastroscopy, a doctor inserts a long tube through your mouth to your stomach.

Ms. Smith: Is it painful?

Hyoja: No, it's 5) ______________ uncomfortable when you swallow the tube, but we'll give you some medicine to anesthetize your throat, so it won't 6) ______________ at all. Once the tube is in, the doctor can examine your esophagus, stomach and duodenum. It's best to relax during the test. If you want, we'll give you a sedative to help you relax.

Ms. Smith: I'm nervous 7) ______________, so I think I'd like a sedative. What's a GI series?

Hyoja: Well, an upper GI series is another test for your stomach and duodenum. In this test you drink some barium sulfate which coats your stomach so that the 8) ______________ of your stomach can be seen on an X-ray. Then the technician takes a lot of X-ray photographs. A lower GI series is a barium enema. In this case the barium is put into your colon by enema. The lining of your colon and rectum can be seen on X-rays.

한글 번역판 참조(133P)

Ms. Smith: Do I 9) ________________ any other tests?

Hyoja: Well, we'll check your blood and blood pressure evey day and I'd like you to 10) ____________________ twice a day. After your doctor sees the results of your tests, she may decide to do some others.

■ The Next Day

Hyoja: You're going to have your lower GI series 11) ____________________.
Today you can't have any solid food; we will give you a liquid meal for breakfast, lunch and dinner, such as broth and rice gruel. Please don't eat anything besides what you are served.

Ms. Smith: What is rice gruel?

Hyoja: It's rice cooked with a lot of water for a long time until it's very soft.

Ms. Smith: I see. Do I need to take a laxative?

Hyoja: Yes, you do. 12) ________________ these 2 tablets at 9 pm and then please don't eat or drink anything after that.

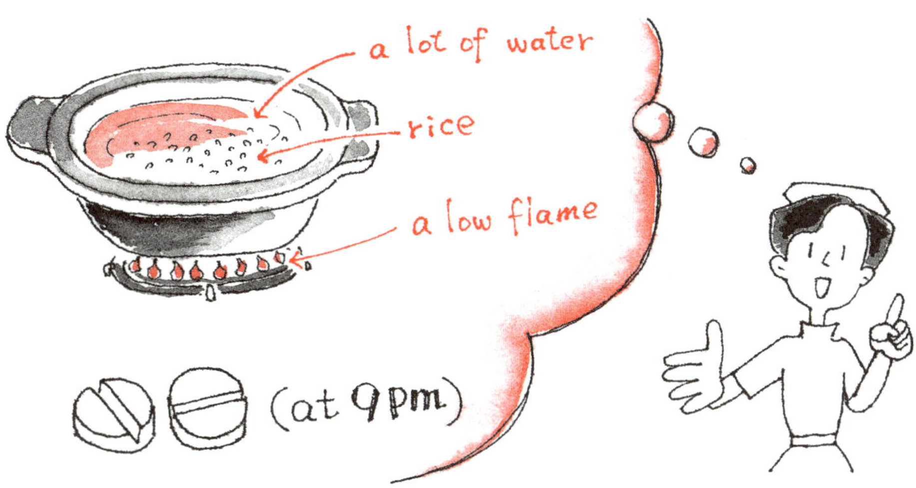

Medical Terms - Tests

Biopsy	생검
blood pressure test	혈압측정
blood specimen collection(blood test)	혈액채취(혈액검사)
CAT(CT) scan(computerized axial tomography)	전산화단층촬영술
colonoscopy	대장내시경
cystoscopy	방광내시경
ECG, EKCG(electrocardiogram, electrocardiography)	심전도
EEG(electroencephalogram, electroencephalography)	뇌파검사
endoscopy	내시경
eye test	시력검사
fecal occult blood test	대변잠혈검사
gastroscopy	위내시경
hearing test	청력검사
laparoscopy	복강경검사
lower GI series(barium enema)	하부 소화기계 조영술 (바륨 관장)
lung function	폐기능검사
mammogram	유방촬영술
MRI(magnetic resonance imaging)	자기공명영상
Pap test, Pap smear(uterine cancer screening)	팝도말검사(자궁암 검사)
RI(radioisotope scan)	방사선 동위원소 검사
spinal tap(lumbar puncture)	요추 천자
sputum test	객담검사
stool test	대변검사
thermography	체열촬영술
ultrasound(echogram, echography)	초음파
upper GI series(barium meal)	상부 소화기계 조영술 (바륨식)
urinalysis(urine test)	소변검사
X-ray	엑스레이

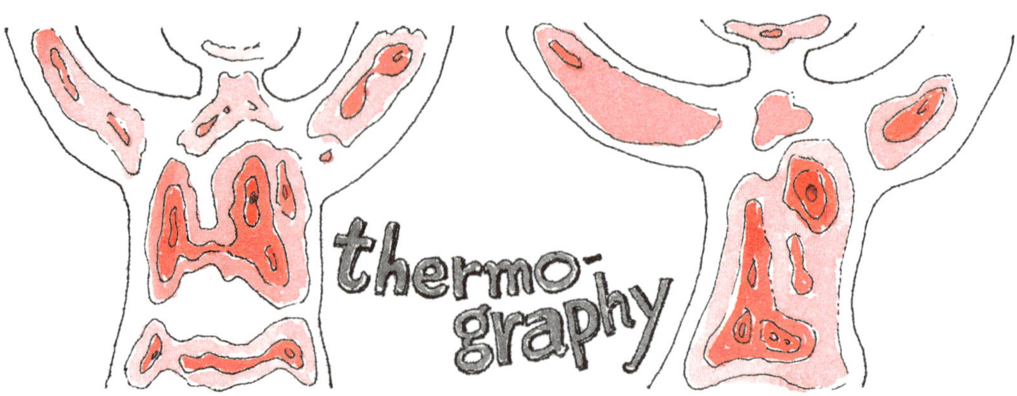

Activity 4: Medical Tests Crossword Puzzle

무슨 검사일까요?

52페이지의 힌트를 참고로 하여 아래의 공란을 채우세요.

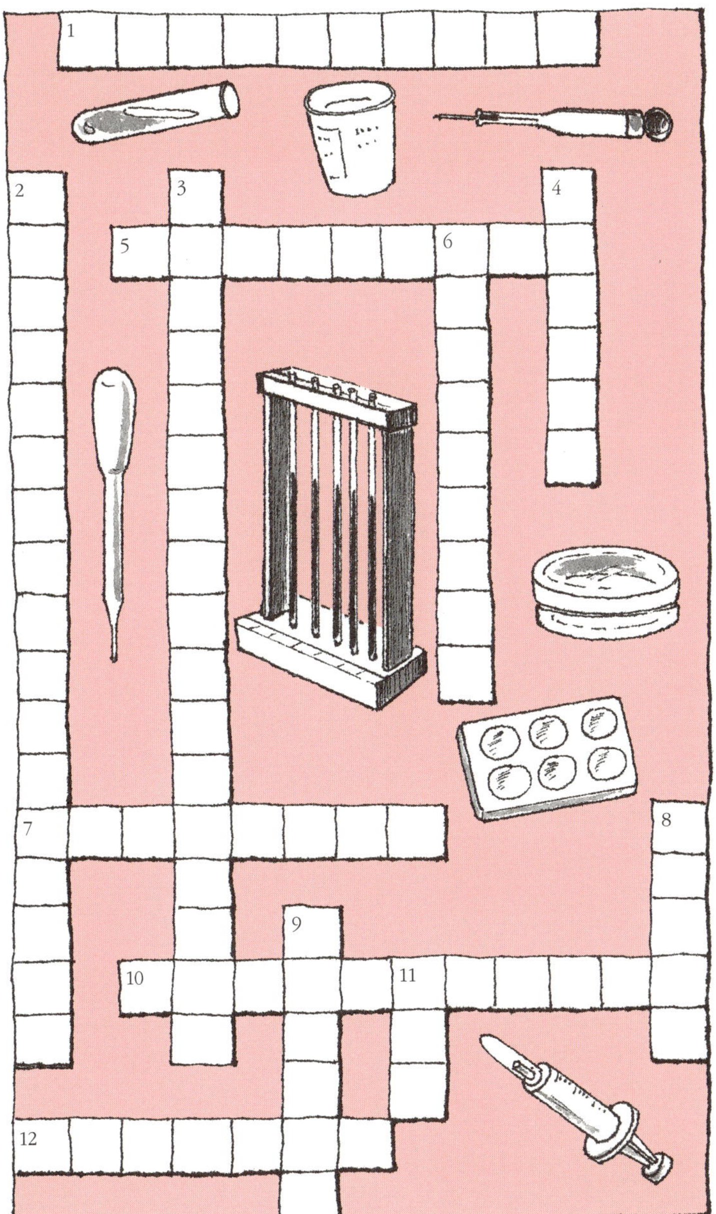

한글 번역판 참조(134P)

ACROSS

1. For this test, the patient puts a sample of urine into a cup which is then tested.
5. In this test, a sample of blood in taken from a person's vein.
7. Also called echography, echo or ultrasound, in this test, sound waves are passed into the body to find abnormalities.
10. In this test, a substance called barium sulfate is inserted by enema. Next, a lot of X-ray pictures of the colon and rectum are taken.
12. In this test, a doctor checks a person's vision.

DOWN

2. In this test, blood pressure cuff is wrapped around the patient's upper arm to check his/her blood pressure.
3. Also called EKG, in this test, a doctor attaches electrodes to a person's chest, wrists and ankles to check the heart.
4. In this test, pictures of sections of the body can be made using computerized tomography.
6. In this test, a doctor inserts a long this tube into a person's body. The doctor can examine the inside of the body, take a photograph or take a tissue sample.
8. A test in which radiation is used to make a picture of the inside of the body, such as the bones.
9. In this test, a doctor removes a small piece of body tissue or some fluid to examine it for abnormalities under a microscope.
11. In this test, the patient is put into a long hollow machine and then magnetic waves are passed through the person's body. In this way a picture of the inside of a person's body can be made. This test is also called Magnetic Resonance Imaging.

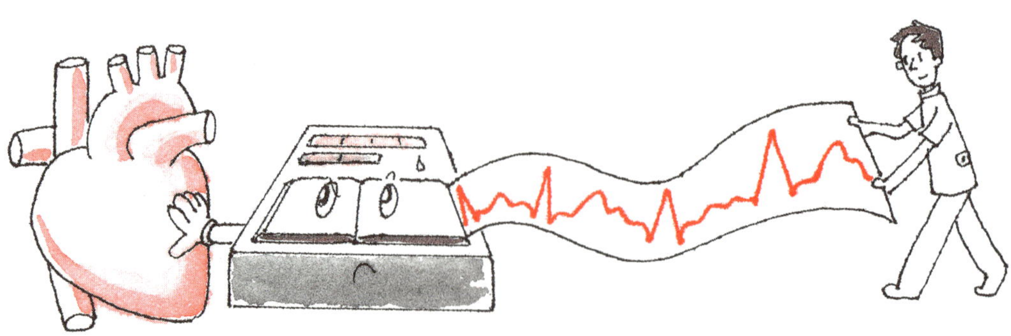

한글 번역판 참조(135P)

Activity 5: Role Play

검사 순서

2인 1조가 되어, 간호사역(A)과 환자역을 정하십시오. 간호사역인 사람은 카드에 적힌 대로 영어로 검사순서를 실연하고, 환자역인 사람은 그 지시에 따르십시오. 끝나면 역할을 바꾸어, 이번에는 간호사(B)의 카드를 사용하여 연습합니다. 시간이 있으면 서로 A, B 양쪽 검사를 연습해 봅시다.

Role Card A-Nurse; Taking a Blood Sample

Read the instructions below several times until you understand; then act out the role play with your partner.

You would like to take a blood sample from your patient. Prepare your syringe and vacuum tube. Tell the patient to sit down and put her arm on the armrest. Tell your patient to make a fist. Tie a tourniquet around the patient's arm. Wipe the patient's arm with cotton soaked in alcohol. Remove the cover from the needle. Tell the patient, "It will sting a little." Insert the needle into the patient's vein. Push in the vacuum tube so the blood flows into the tube. Tell the Patient to open her fist. Remove the tourniquet from the patient's arm. Place alcohol-soaked cotton over the puncture and remove the needle. Tape a band-aid on the puncture. Tell the patient to apply pressure for a few minutes.

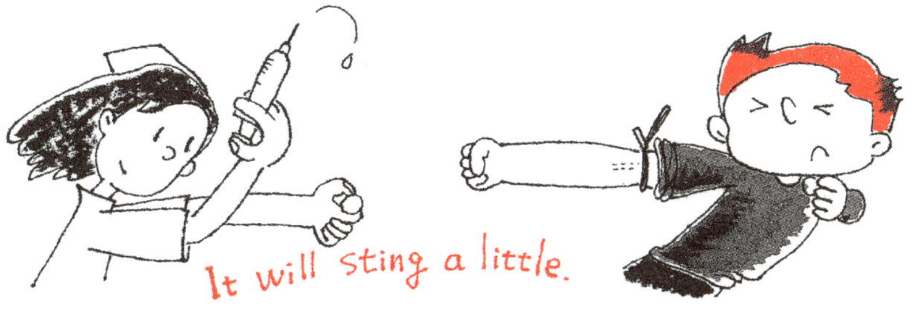

한글 번역판 참조(135P)

Role Card B-Nurse: Checking Respiration and Pulse

Read the instructions below several times until you understand: then act out the role play with your partner.

You would like to check your patient's respiration and pulse. Prepare your stethoscope. Tell your patient you would like to check his respiration and pulse. Ask your patient to sit up(down) and raise his shirt. Put the stethoscope against our patient's chest. Tell the patient to breathe(inhale) deeply and hold his breath. Tell the patient to exhale. Tell the patient to inhale and exhale several times as you listen to different spots. Next, tell the patient to turn around and put the stethoscope against the patient's back. Tell the patient to inhale and exhale several times as you listen to different spots. When you finish, tell the patient to pull down his shirt. Next, tell the patient you are going to take his pulse. Put your fingers against his wrist and time his pulse. When you are finished, tell the patient you are finished.

Activity 6: Game-Three Hints

검사명 대기

이것은 그룹(가능하면 4인 1조)으로 하는 carta(트럼프)게임입니다. 2조의 카드 중, Medical Tests Cards(정답 카드)는 겉을 위로 하여 책상 위에 펼쳐 놓습니다. Three Hints Cards(문제 카드)는 각자에게 나누어 주고, 각각 자기 앞에 엎어 놓습니다.

최초의 사람이 갖고 있는 카드를 1장 빼서, 거기에 적혀 있는 3가지 힌트를 한가지씩 소리내어 읽습니다. 그 외의 사람들은 대답 카드 중에서 바른 검사명이 적혀 있는 것을 찾아냅니다. 카드는 찾은 사람의 것이 됩니다. 이번에는 다음 사람이 문제를 읽습니다. 이와 같이 순서에 따라 하고, 마지막에 가장 많은 카드를 가지고 있는 사람이 이깁니다.

UNIT 6

You're going to have a baby!

한글 번역판 참조(136P)

Activity 1: Listening Practice

CD 17

Listen to the conversations and choose the correct answers.

1. What does the patient want?
   a) She wants to have an abortion.
   b) She wants a pregnancy test.
   c) She wants a contraceptive.

2. How does Sarah know she's pregnant?
   a) She missed her period.
   b) Her doctor gave her a pregnancy test.
   c) Her home pregnancy test was positive.

3. How old was the patient when she started menstruating?
   a) She was 17 years old. b) 2 weeks ago.
   c) She was 12 years old.

4. What kind of test does the patient want?
   a) She wants a pregnancy test. b) She wants an HIV test.
   c) She wants a herpes test.

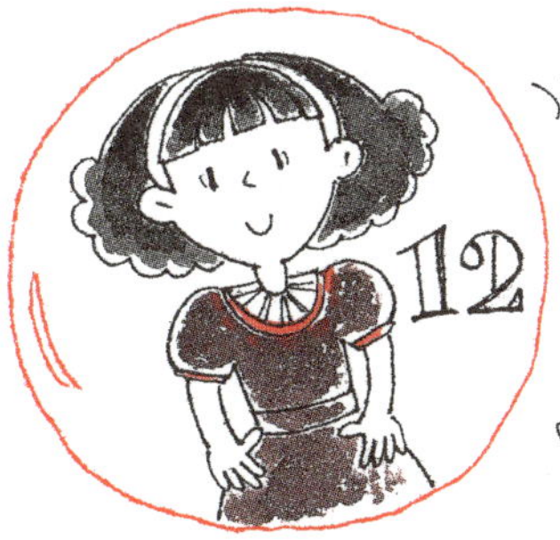

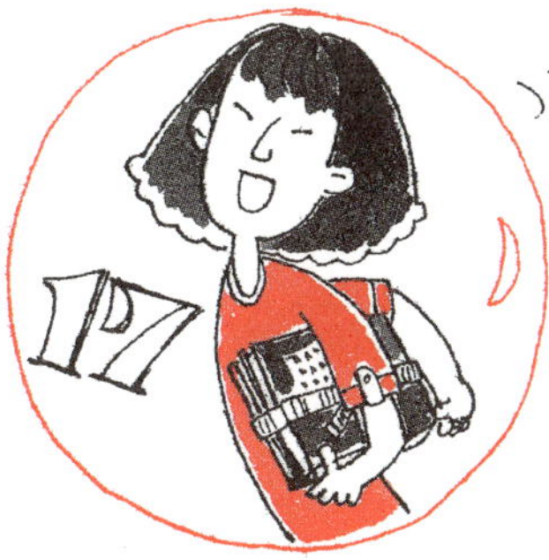

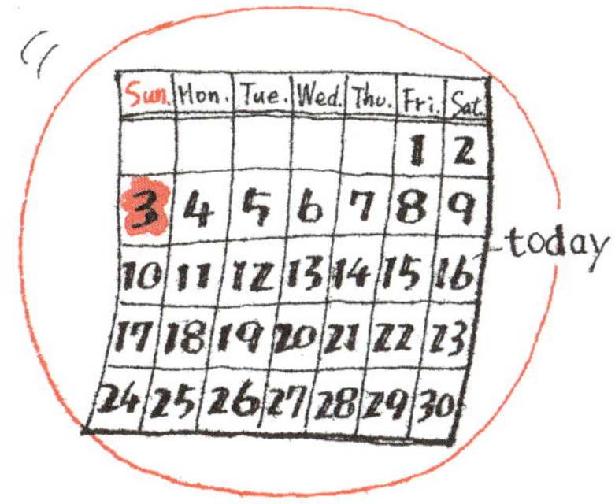

Activity 2: Checkpoint

CD 1

산부인과외래

1. 무슨 일로 오셨습니까?

What's the purpose of your visit?

임신반응(자궁암) 검사를 받으러 왔습니다.

I want a pregnancy(Pap) test.

에치아이브이(매독, 임질, 헤르프스) 검사를 받으러 왔습니다.

I want an HIV(syphilis gonorrhea, herpes) test.

피임약을 받으러 왔습니다(자궁내장치술을 받으러 왔습니다).

I want birth control pills(an IUD).

호르몬 대체 요법을 받으러 왔습니다.

I want hormone replacement therapy.

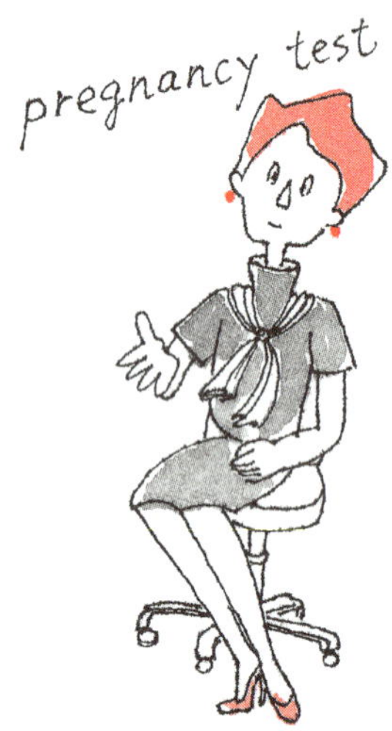

2. 언제가 마지막 월경일입니까?

When was your last period?

3. 월경은 규칙적입니까 아니면 불규칙적입니까?

Are your periods regular or irregular?

4. 초경을 언제 하셨습니까?

When did you start menstruating?

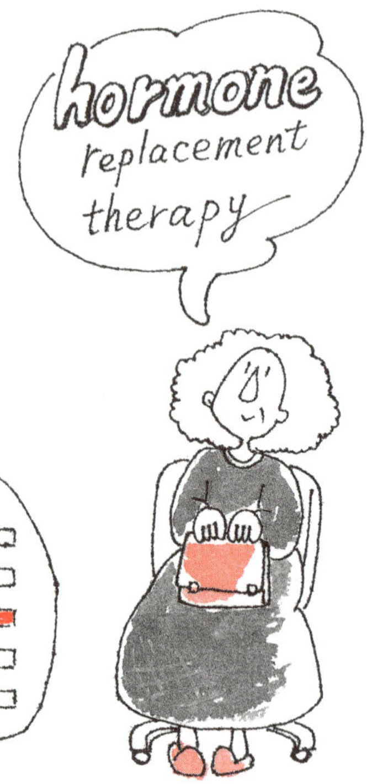

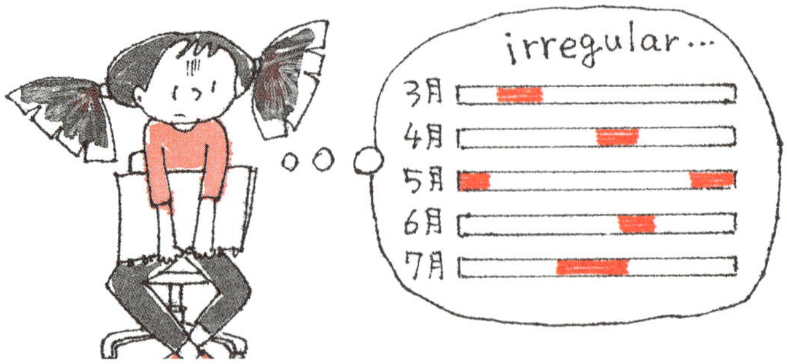

5. 어떤 피임법(피임제, 가족계획)을 사용하시나요?
What kind of birth control(contraceptive, family planning) do you use?
  콘돔(자궁내장치, 피임약)을 사용합니다.
  I use condoms(an IUD, birth control pills).

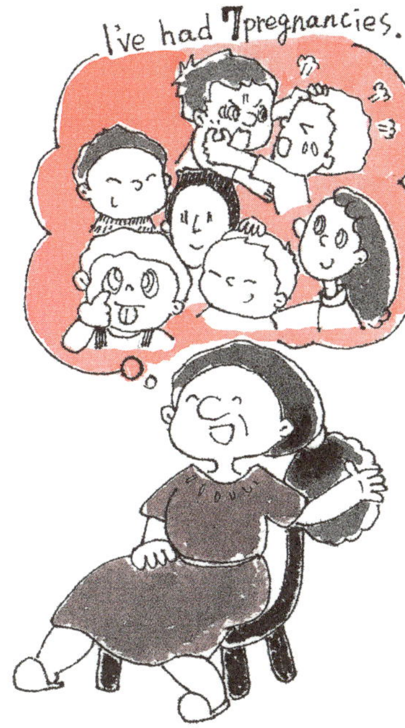

6. 임신을 몇 번 해보셨습니까?
How many pregnancies have you had?

7. 임신 했을 때마다 출산을 하셨습니까?
Have they all resulted in live births?
  예 그렇습니다./아니오, 한 번은 유산되었습니다.
  Yes, they have./No, I had one miscarriage.

8. 사산아를 낳으신 적이 있습니까?
Have you had any stillbirths?

9. 자연분만을 하셨습니까, 아니면 제왕절개술을 받으셨습니까?
Did you have a normal birth or a cesarean?
  첫 분만은 자연분만이었고, 두 번째 분만은 제왕절개술이었습니다.
  My first delivery was normal; the second was by cesarean section.

10. 유산이나 낙태(임신중절술)의 경험이 있습니까?
Have you had any miscarriages or abortions?

11. 언제 월경이 멈추었습니까?/언제 폐경이 시작되었습니까?
When did you stop menstruating?/When did you start menopause?

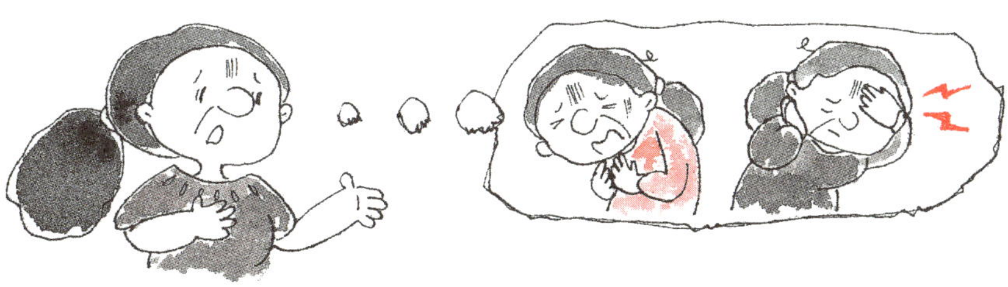

한글 번역판 참조(137P)

Activity 3: Dialog

CD 19

Listen to the dialog and fill in the missing words.

■ At the Maternity Clinic

Dal: Congratulations! I heard you're going 1) ______________.

Ms. Fisher: Thank you. The doctor said my expected date of delivery is September 7th.

Dal: This booklet is a Maternal and Child Health Handbook. In Korea, we say "Maternal pocket book" 2)______________ every time you visit. This will be a record of your pregnancy. And after your baby is born, it will be a record of your baby's health and inoculations.

Ms. Fisher: What 3) ______________ will the doctor do when I come for my check-ups?

Dal: She'll check your blood pressure, urine, and weight gain. She'll also do an internal examination and an echogram to check the development of the fetus.

■ 34 Weeks Later

Dal: How far apart are your contractions?

Ms. Fisher: 4) ______________.

Dal: Please change into your gown and we'll go to the 5) ______________ room.

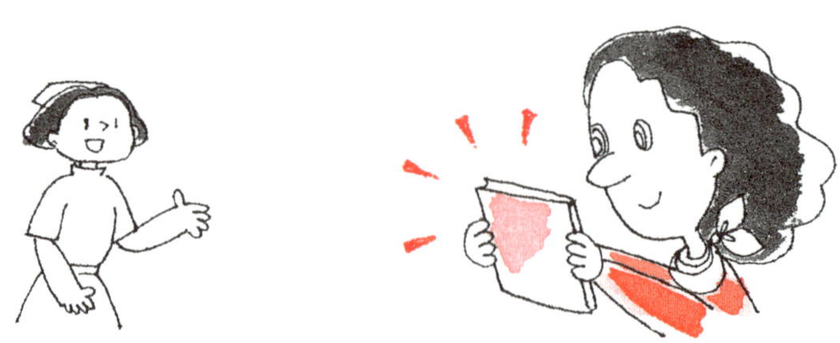

한글 번역판 참조(138P)

■ In the Labor Room

Dal: You are fully dilated. 6) ______________ the delivery room.

Dr. Sunyoung: Your baby's head is crowning. Push, push. OK. Now, breathe. Breathe again. OK, now, push, 7) ______________, one more time. There you go. You have a beautiful baby girl.

Dal: Let me clean her up and then you can hold her. Here you are.

■ After the Delivery-Mrs. Fisher's Room

Dal: You can breast-feed your baby every time she cries. Please weigh her 8) ______________ breast-feeding and write the weight here. After feeding her, please change her diaper.

Ms. Fisher: I don't have too much milk yet and 9) ______________ yellow.

Dal: The first breast milk is called "colostrum". It's very 10) ______________

■ Day of Discharge

Dal: Your baby will 11) ______________ of the time. But she may wake up frequently during the night for feeding. Be sure that you get enough rest.

Ms. Fisher: When do I have to come back for a check-up?

Dal: Please come back in 4 weeks. But 12) ______________ like a fever, diarrhea, breathing difficulties, convulsions or jaundice, call the hospital immediately.

Ms. Fisher: OK. Thank you very much for all your help.

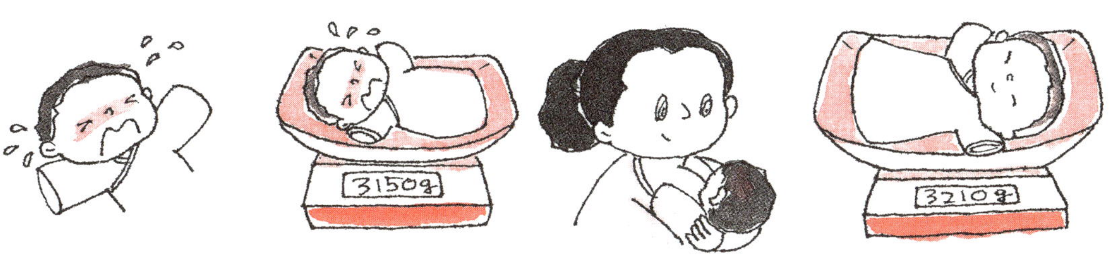

UNIT 6

Medical Terms - Obstetrics & Gynecology

Abortion	유산
afterbirth	출생 후
AIDS(acquired immunodeficiency syndrome)	에이즈(후천성 면역 결핍증)
amniocentesis	양수천자검사
anesthesia	마취
Apgar sore	아프가 점수
birth control	산아 제한
birth control pills(the Pill)	경구 피임약
breech presentation	둔위
cell	세포
cervix	자궁경부
cervical cancer	자궁경부암
cesarean section	제왕절개술
circumcision	포경수술
colostrum	초유
contraceptive	피임제
contraction(s)	수축
convulsion(s)	경련
crowning	배림(머리출현)
delivery	분만
delivery room	분만실
development(of fetus)	(태아)발달
D&C(dilatation & curettage)	디엔씨(자궁경관확장소파술)
dilate	확장하다
echogram	초음파
eclampsia	자간증
effacement	자궁경부소실
embryo	배아
emesis(vomiting)	구토
epidural block	경막외차단 마취
episiotomy	회음절개술
expected date of delivery	분만 예정일
face presentation	안위(얼굴 태위)
fallopian tube	나팔관
fetal monitoring	태아감시
fetus	태아
forceps	겸자
gonorrhea	임질
gynecologist	부인과의사
herpes	헤르페스
HIV(human immunodeficiency virus)	에치아이브이(사람면역결핍바이러스)
home pregnancy test	가정용임신반응검사
hot flash	작열감(폐경기)
HRT(hormone replacement therapy)	에치알티(호르몬 대체 요법)

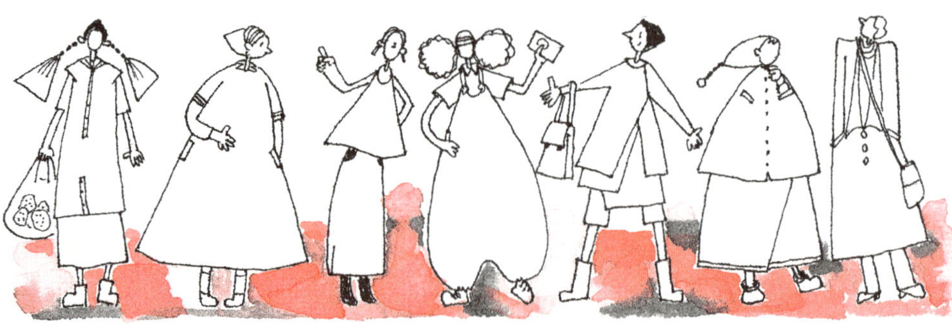

Medical Terms - Obstetrics & Gynecology

intercourse	성교	ovulate	배란
painful intercourse	성교통	Pap test, Pap smear	팝 도말검사
Internal examination(exam)	내진	period(monthly period)	월경(월경주기)
IUD(intrauterine device)	자궁내 장치	miss one's period	월경을 거르다
Jaundice	황달	placenta	태반
labor	분만	PMS(premenstrual syndrome)	피엠에스(월경전 증후군)
labor pain	산통	postpartum blues	산후 우울증
labor room	분만대기실	pre-eclampsia	자간전증
live birth	생존출생	pregnancy test	임신반응검사
Menopause	폐경	premature test	조산
menstruate	월경	rectal examination	직장 검사
painful menstruation	월경통	STD(sexually transmitted disease)	에스티디(성행위 전염병)
midwife	조산사	stillbirth	사산
miscarriage	유산	syphilis	매독
morning sickness	입덧	trimester	(임신)3분기
myoma of the uterus	자궁근종	umbilical cord	탯줄
neonate, newborn	신 생아	uterus(womb) vacuum extraction	자궁 진공 분만
normal birth	자연분만	vagina	질
obstetrician	산과의사	vaginal examination	질 내진
organ	장기	weight gain	체중 증가

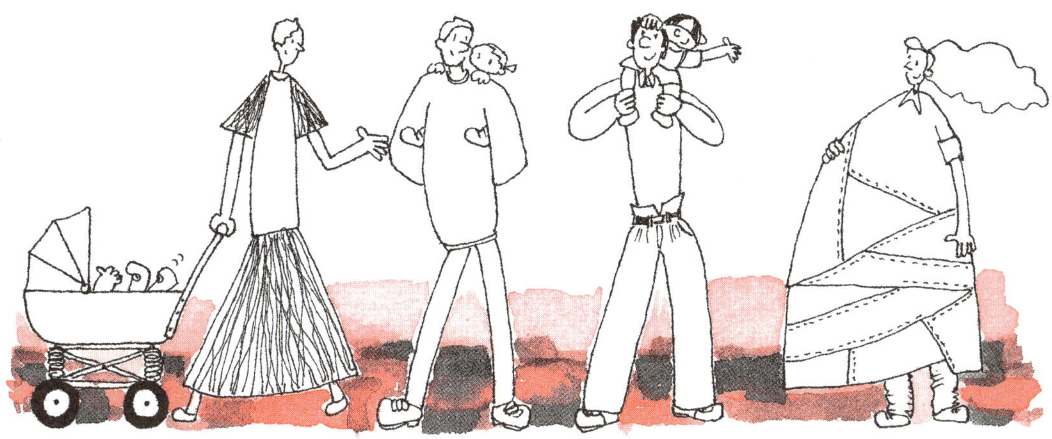

한글 번역판 참조(139P)

Activity 4: Game - Your Childhood

어떤 아기였는가?

클라스메이트 3명에게 유아기의 추억에 관하여 영어로 인터뷰합시다. 아래 표에 상대방의 이름과 대답을 기입하십시오. 자기 그룹 이외의 사람에게 물어 보도록 하세요.

When you were a child···	Name:	Name:	Name:
1. Did you have a "security blanket"? What was it?			
2. What was your "comfort food" when you were sick?			
3. What was your favorite toy or book?			
4. Did you go to nursery school or kindergarten? From what age?			
5. Did you have a pet? What was it?			
6. Who was your best friend?			
7. Did you have any serious injury? What was it?			
8. Were you ever hospitalized?			

한글 번역판 참조(139P)

Activity 5: Role Play

산부인과 예진표

2인 1조가 되어, 간호사역(A)와 환자역(B)를 정하십시오. 간호사는 환자에게 질문하고, 아래 서류에 기입합니다. 끝나면 역할을 바꾸어, 이번에는 환자(C)와 간호사(A)의 카드를 사용하여 연습합니다.

Role Card A-Nurse

Your patient is a foreigner who can't understand Korean. Ask your patient the questions to help her fill in the form.

성명 ______________________ 연령 __________

초경연령 ______________________

최종월경 ______________________

월경주기 규칙/불규칙 ______________ 일형

폐경 예/아니오 폐경연령 ______________

임신횟수 ________

분만횟수 ________

1. 정상분만/제왕절개
2. 정상분만/제왕절개
3. 정상분만/제왕절개

어린이의 연령 성별 ______________________

통상의 피임방법 ______________________

진료의 목적 ______________________

주요증상 ______________________

언제부터 ______________________

기타 증상 ______________________

한글 번역판 참조(140P)

Role Card B-Patient; Sylvia Franco, 55-year-old female

You started menstruation when you were 13 years old. Your periods are very irregular; your last period was 3 months ago. You have a period every few months.

You have 3 children, 2 sons, 24 and 26 years old and 1 daughter, 16 years old. You delivered your first 2 children by normal delivery and your daughter by cesarean section.

You use a condom as birth control.

You want to see the doctor about getting hormone replacement therapy. Your problem is that intercourse is painful. You've had this problem for about 3 years. Your other symptoms are hot flashes and cold sweats.

Role Card C-Patient; Julia May Bookman, 24-year-old female

You had your first period when you were $11\frac{1}{2}$years old. Your periods are regular, every 28 days. Your last period was 2 weeks ago.

You were pregnant once, but had a miscarriage in your 5th week. You don't have any children.

Now, you are using a condom as birth control, but you would like to change to the Pill. You want to see the doctor about getting the Pill.

You have no other problems or symptoms.

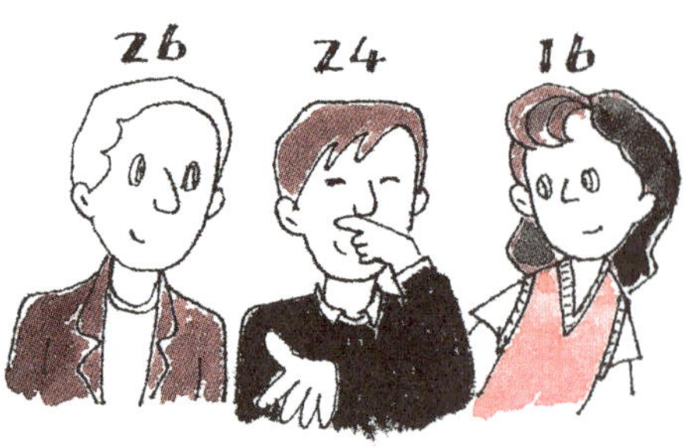

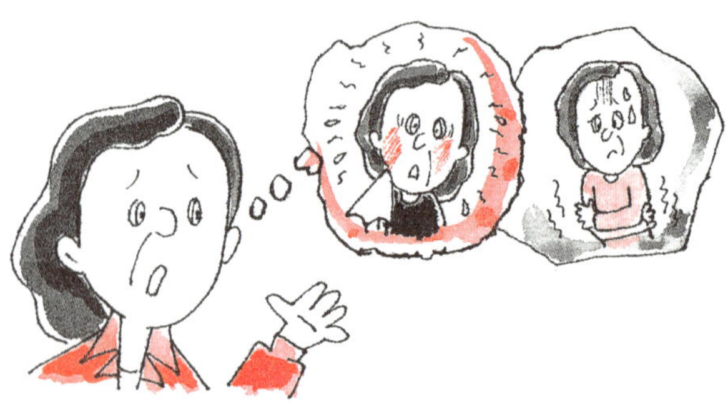

Activity 6: Crossword Puzzle-Having a baby!

임신과 출산

공란에는 임신·출산에 곤한 18가지 용어가 들어갑니다. 다음 페이지의 힌트를 읽고 답하세요.

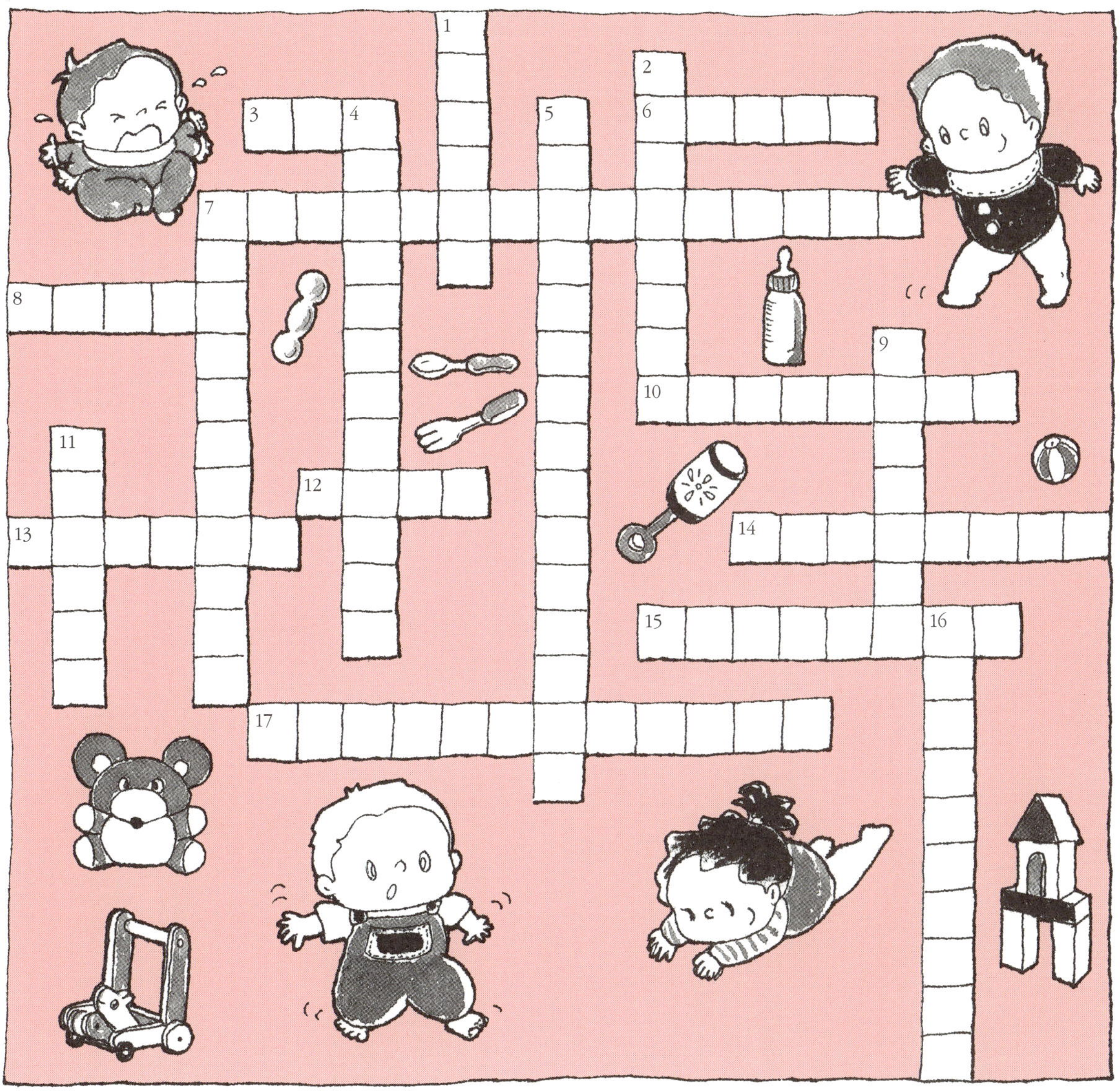

UNIT 6

한글 번역판 참조(141P)

ACROSS

3. A procedure for doing an abortion by dilating the cervix and scraping the uterus.
6. The process of pushing out the fetus.
7. The feeling of nausea that many pregnant women experience in the early part of pregnancy.
8. The baby before it is born.
10. Artificial ending of a pregnancy.
12. Women take this as one form of birth control.
13. The lower end of the uterus, between the uterus and vagina.
14. Giving birth to a baby.
15. A test in which a doctor removes some cells from a women's cervix to check then for cancer.
17. A way couples use to prevent becoming pregnant, such as a condom.

DOWN

1. A woman's sexual organ through which a baby is born in a normal delivery.
2. An organ lining the uterus, connected to the fetus by the umbilical cord and providing food for the fetus.
4. During birth, a woman experiences these. They help push out the fetus.
5. Delivery of a baby by cutting open the abdomen.
7. A spontaneous(happening by itself) ending of a pregnancy.
9. A nurse who is specially trained to deliver babies.
11. The part of a woman's body in which the fetus grows.
16. A test give to a newborn to check its physical condition.

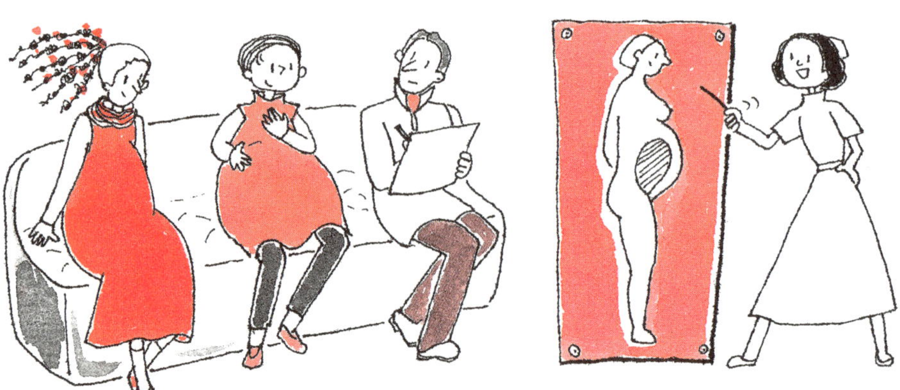

UNIT 7

My baby has a fever.

한글 번역판 참조(142P)

Activity 1: Listening Practice

CD 20

Listen to the conversations and choose the correct answers.

1. How long has Mary been sick?
   a) 38.7°　　b) for 3 days　　c) for 1 day

2. When did Howard have his first DPT inoculation?
   a) three days ago　　b) over a year ago　　c) last week

3. What is the problem with Ms. Ryan's daughter?
   a) She's vomiting.　　b) She hit her head.　　c) She's crying too much.

4. What vaccination does the father want for his son?
   a) Diphtheria, pertussis, tetanus
   b) Japanese encephalitis
   c) Measles, mumps, and rubella

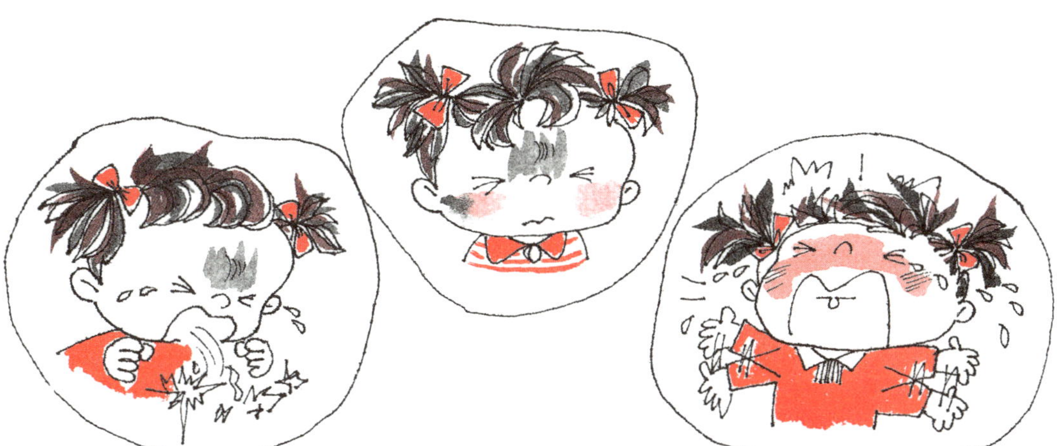

Activity 2: Checkpoint

CD

예방접종을 설명한다.

1. 우리 아기는 어떤 예방 접종을 받아야 합니까?

What inoculations(vaccinations, vaccine) should my baby get?

디피티(소아마비, 풍진, 홍역, 이하선염, 수두, 결핵) 예방 접종을 받아야 합니다.

Your baby needs to get a DPT(polio, rubella, measles, mumps, chicken-pox, BCG) inoculation.

2. 그(그녀)는 언제 예방 접종을 받아야 합니까?

When should he(she) get the inoculatioin?

2개월과 1세 사이에 받아야 합니다.

Between 2 months and 1 year.

4개월 때 받아야 합니다.

At 4 months.

3. 그(그녀)는 그 예방접종주사를 몇 번 맞아야 합니까?

How many time does he(she) need to have the inoculation?

세 번(4주 간격으로) 맞아야 합니다.

He(she) needs to get it 3 times(at 4-week intervals).

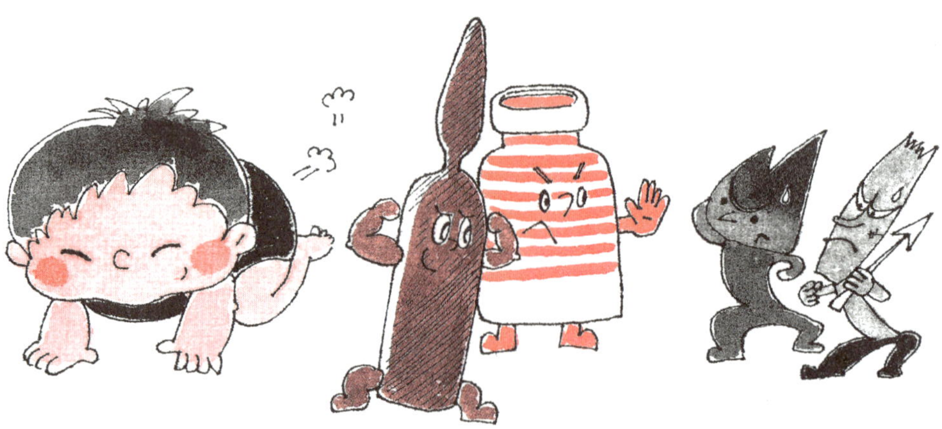

4. 제 아들(딸)은 추가 접종을 받아야 합니까?

Does my son(daughter) need to get a booster?

예, 그(그녀)는 첫 접종 후 일 년 후에 추가 접종을 받아야 합니다.

Yes, he(she) needs a booster 1 year after the original inoculation.

그(그녀)는 4, 5년 마다 추가 접종을 받아야 합니다.

He(she) needs a booster every 4 to 5 years.

5. 제 아들(딸)은 어디서 예방접종 주사를 맞을 수 있습니까?

Where can my son(daughter) get the inoculations?

그(그녀)는 보건소에서 예방접종 주사를 맞을 수 있습니다.

He(She) can get some inculcations at the public health center.

다른 예방 접종 주사는 병원이나 클리닉에서 맞습니다.

Other inoculations are given at a hospital or a clinic.

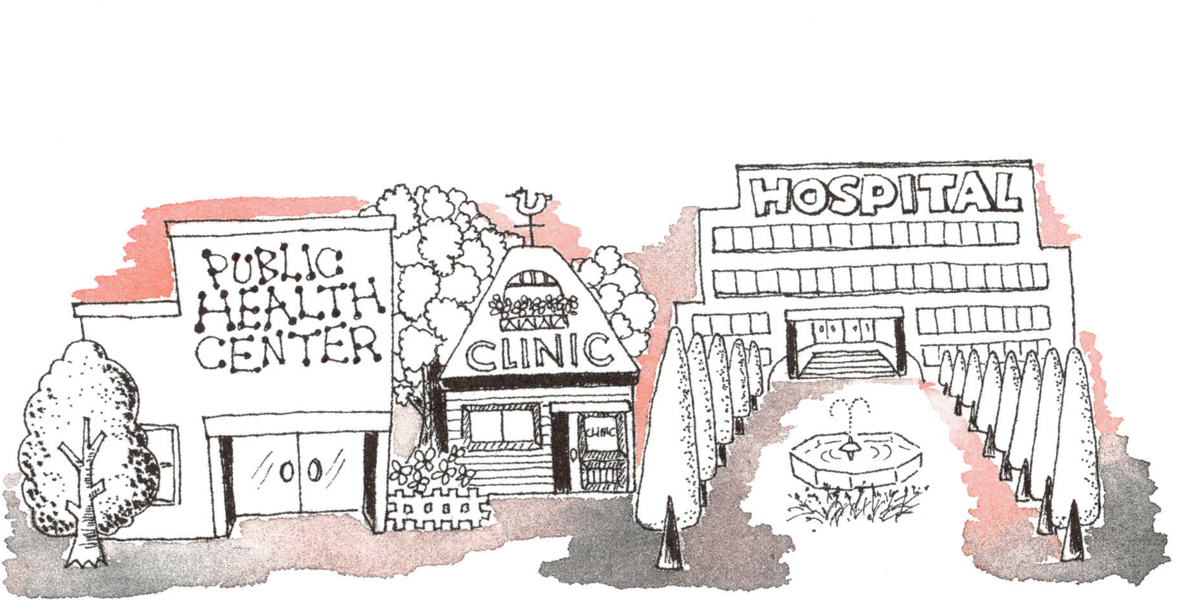

한글 번역판 참조(143P)

Activity 3: Dialog

CD

Listen to the dialog and fill in the missing words.

■ **At the Pediatrician's**

Hyojin: Kim Dohyun?

Mrs. Aram: Yes. 1) ________________ Dohyun.

Hyojin: How old is your son?

Mrs. Aram: He's 9 months old.

Hyojin: What seems 2) ________________________________?

Mrs. Aram: He's cranky and lethargic. He's been touching 3) ____________ a lot.

Hyojin: Let's check his temperature. Please put this thermometer 4) ________ ________________. Has he had any medical problems before?

Mrs. Aram: Well, he often seems to have a cold. He had roseola when he was about 3 months old.

Hyojin: Does Kim 5) ______________________, especially drug allergies?

Mrs. Aram: I don't think he's allergic to any drugs, but he's allergic to eggs.

Hyojin: OK. Let's see. He 6) __________________________. His temperature is 38.5°. Plese wait; the doctor will see you soon.

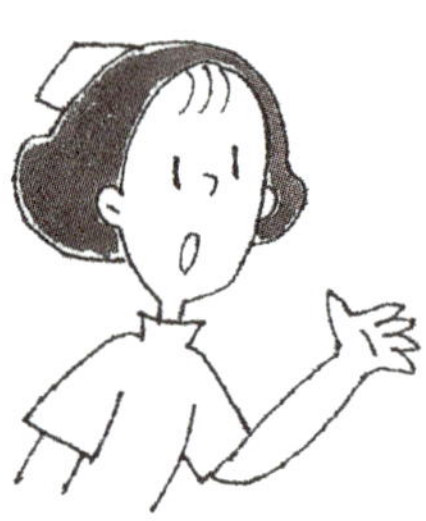

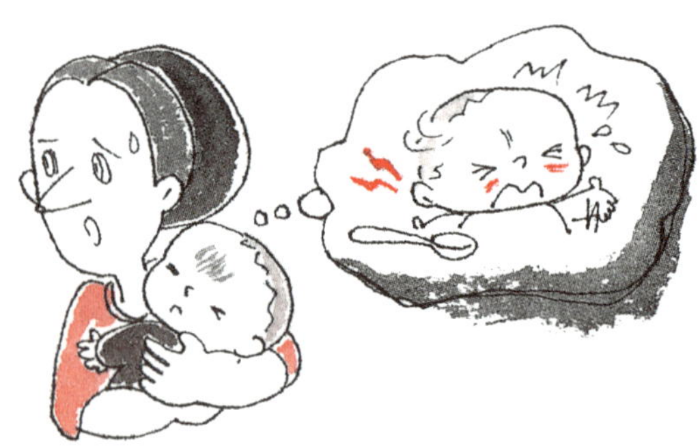

한글 번역판 참조(144P)

■ Later

Mrs. Aram: The doctor said Dohyun 7) ______________ an ear infection. She said she'd give me some antibiotics and if the infection didn't clear up she said I'd better take Dohyun to an ENT specialist.

Hyojin: Here's Dohyun's medication. This is an antibiotic. It's a powder, so 8) ______________ with some juice. Please give it to him three times a day after meals. And this yellow powder is for fever. Please give it to him if his temperature is higher than 38°. 9) ______________ or problems, please don't hesitate to call.

Mrs. Aram: Thank you. Actually, I have some questions about Dohyun's inoculations. He had DPT, Polio and BCG when he was about 5 months old. 10) ______________ does he need?

Hyojin: Well, he should have DPT 3 times, polio twice and BCG once.

Mrs. Aram: I see. Are there any 11) ______________ he needs?

Hyojin: He should get rubella, measles, mumps and chickenpox vaccinations, but those are given after he is one year old. Then there's the inoculations for Japanese encephalitis.

Mrs. Aram: 12) ______________________?

Hyojin: It's a disease carried by mosquitoes. Here, I can give you a schedule of inoculations in English.

Mrs. Aram: Thank you.

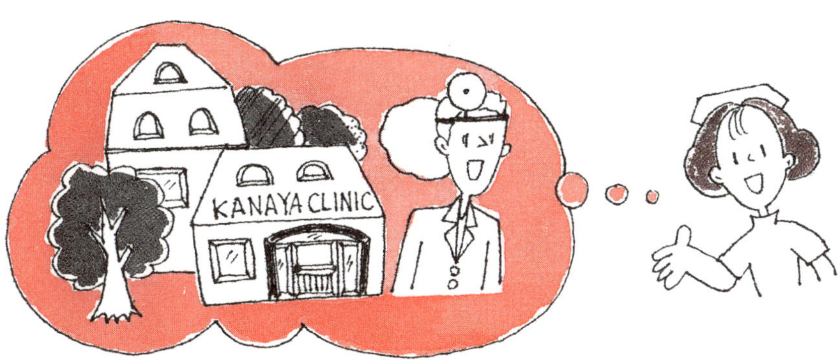

Medical Terms - Vaccinations

예방 접종

접종 종류	횟수	간격	연령
DPT(diphtheria/pertussis/tetanus) 디프테리아, 백일해, 파상풍 booster 추가 접종	3회 1회	3~8주 간격	3~90개월 사이 최종 DPT 접종으로부터 6개월 이후
DT(diphtheria/tetanus) 디프테리아, 파상풍	1회		11~12세
Polio 소아마비	2회	6주 간격	3~90개월 사이
MMR(measles/mumps/rubella) 홍역 / 이하선염 / 풍진 booster 추가 접종	1회 1회		12~24개월 사이 만4~6세 사이
Chickenpox 수두	1회		1세 이후
BCG 비씨지(결핵)	1회		태어나서 6개월 사이

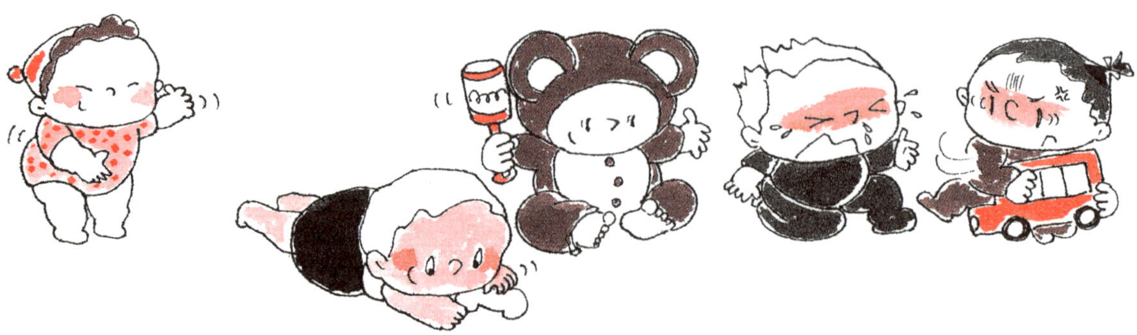

Medical Terms - Childhood Health Problems

Disease, Disordrs

ADHD(attention deficit hyperactivity disorder)	주의력 결핍과 과잉행동장애
atopic dermatitis	아토피 피부염
autism	자폐증
bronchitis	기관지염
colic	복통,산통
convulsion(s)	경련
croup	크룹(급성후두기관염)
Down's syndrome	다운 증후군
ear infection(otitis media)	중이염
food poisoning	식중독
gastroenteritis	위장염
hydrocephalus	뇌수종
impetigo	농가진
Kawasaki disease(MCLS, mucotaneous lymph node syndrome)	가와사키병(MCLS, 피부점막림프절증후군)
mental retardation	정신지체장애
pinworm	요충
rheumtic fever	류마티스열
roseaola(-infantum)	장미진(영아)
SIDS(sudden infant death syndrome, crib death)	영아 돌연사 증후군
stomatitis	구내염
strep throat	연쇄상 구균성 인후염
shuttering	말더듬
tonsillitis	편도선염
tuberculosis	결핵

Symptoms, Problems

Bed-wetting	소아야뇨증
breathing difficulty	호흡곤란
child abuse	소아학대
choking	질식
cranking	변덕스러움
crying	울음
cyanosis	청색증
dehydration	탈수
diaper rash	기저기 발진
edema	부종
feeding problems	수유 곤란
heat rash	홍색 땀띠
irritability	흥분, 과민
lethargy	기면, 무기력
lice<louse	이<기생성 곤충의 총칭
sleeping problem	수면 장애
swallowed foreign object	이물질 섭취
teething	생치(치아발육)
wheezing	천명

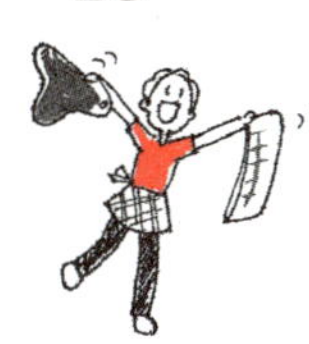

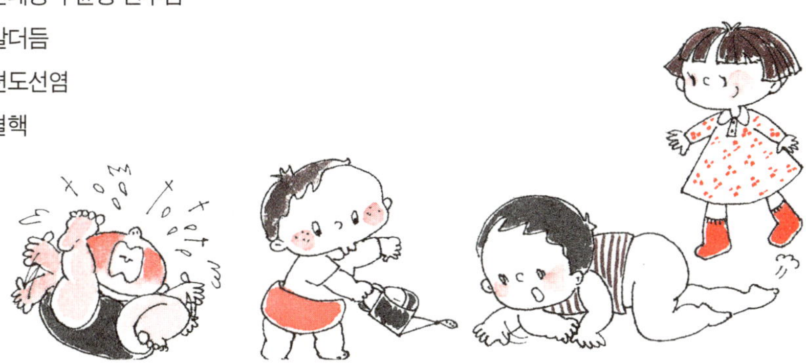

Activity 4: Puzzle-Word Search-Vaccinations

무슨 예방접종을 합니까?

다음 단어를 아래 표 속에서 찾아서 동그라미로 그려 주세요. 3~11의 영어 옆에 접종명을 적어 봅시다.

1. BCG ______________________
2. DPT ______________________
3. PERTUSSIS ______________________
4. RUBELLA ______________________
5. CHICKENPOX ______________________
6. MUMPS ______________________
7. POLIO ______________________
8. TETANUS ______________________
9. DIPHTHERIA ______________________
10. MEASLES ______________________

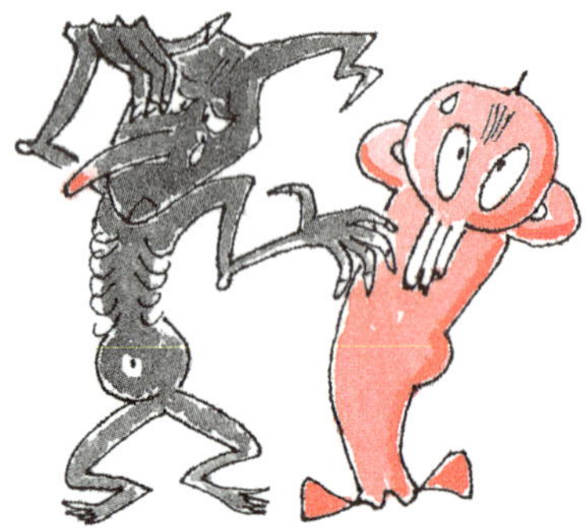

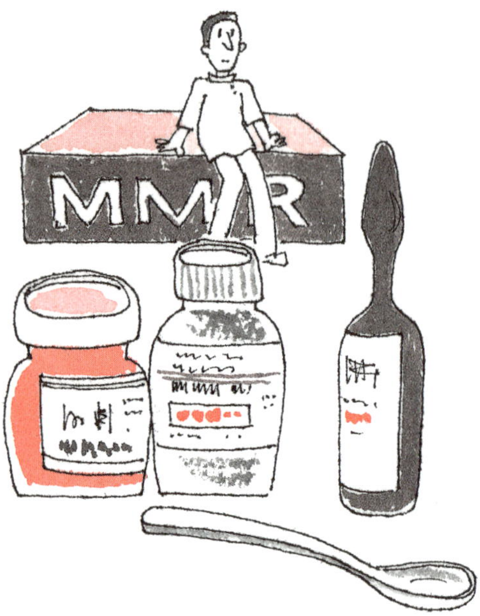

E	M	M	I	P	S	E	L	S	A	E	M
D	N	U	M	O	R	N	U	D	X	O	O
I	P	C	M	R	W	N	E	L	G	I	C
P	S	T	E	P	S	O	D	B	L	H	X
H	I	E	U	P	S	T	I	O	I	H	L
T	S	T	M	Z	H	F	P	C	X	X	F
H	S	A	J	D	O	A	K	O	A	X	X
E	U	N	G	Y	D	E	L	A	X	A	H
R	T	U	P	P	N	C	G	I	G	T	Q
I	R	S	T	P	N	L	J	I	T	C	U
A	E	G	O	F	A	D	W	J	D	I	B
J	P	X	V	A	L	L	E	B	U	R	S

한글 번역판 참조(145P)

Activity 5: Role Play

소아과외래

2인 1조가 되어, 간호사(A)와 소아환자의 부친(C)의 카드를 사용하여 Role Play를 합시다. 다음에 역할을 바꾸어, 간호사(B)와 모친(D)의 카드를 사용하여 연습합시다.

Role Play Card A-Nurse

You are a nurse working in pediatrics. A girl, Susan, comes to your department with her father.

Ask her father questions to fill out the form below.

Tell the girl you will take a sample of her blood. Then tell the father and daughter the doctor will see her quickly.

소아과 예진표

환자성명 ______________ 연령 ________ 남/여

수진이유 ______________________________

통증 유/무 어떤통증 ______________________

통증부위 ______________ 언제부터 ______________

다른증상 ______________________________

기왕력

병명 ______________ 연령 ______________

병명 ______________ 연령 ______________

병명 ______________ 연령 ______________

알레르기 ______________________________

한글 번역판 참조(145P)

Role Play Card B-Nurse

You are a nurse working in pediatrics. A boy, Billy, comes to your department with his mother.

Ask his mother questions to fill out the form below

Ms. Smith asks you what other inoculations he needs. Explain the inoculations he still needs(Hint: use the chart of vaccinations.).

Tell the mother, she must let the doctor know that Billy is allergic to eggs before he gets a measles vaccination.

Tell the mother, if Billy feels sick or has a high fever after the vaccination, she should bring him to the hospital.

예방접종신청서

환자성명 ______________ 연령 ________ 남/여

희망하는 예방접종 ______________________________

체온 ______________________________

병력 병명 ______________ 연령 ________

병명 ______________ 연령 ________

알레르기 ______________________________

희망하는 예방접종 ______________ 연령 ________

______________ ________

______________ ________

______________ ________

______________ ________

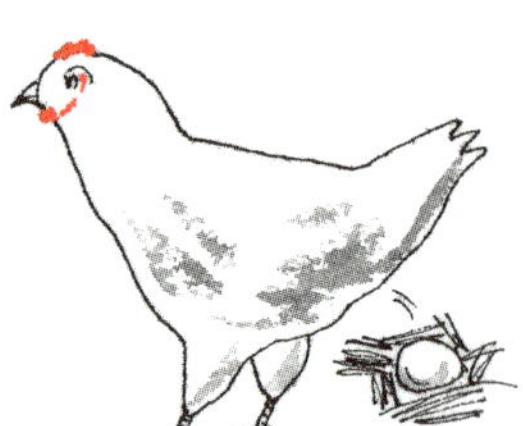

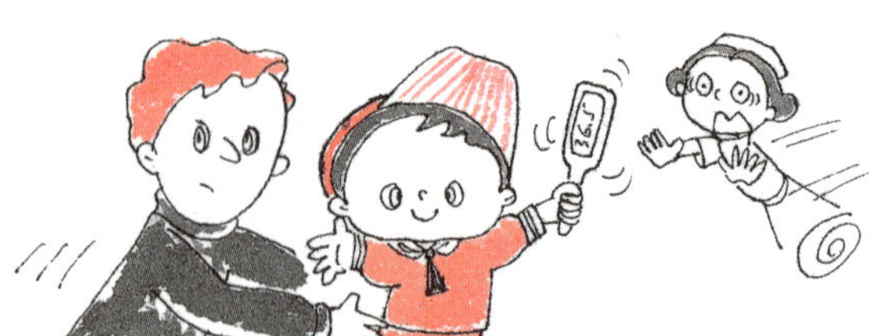

한글 번역판 참조(146P)

Role Card C-Patient' s Father; Mr. Lee

You brought your 11-year-old daughter, Susan Lee, to the hospital because she is feeling sharp and severe pain in her right abdominal area. She's had pain for 2 days. She also feels nauseous and has a fever. Her temperature is 37.8°.

Susan had bronchial pneumonia when she was 5 years old. She's had asthma for about 3 years. She's allergic to penicillin, house dust and mold.

Role Card D-Patient' s Mother; Ms. Smith

You brought your 4-year-old son, Billy Smith, to the hospital because you want him to get a chickenpox vaccination.

He is feeling fine. His temperature is 36.5°.

Billy had roseola when he was 6 months old. He often suffers from ear infections. The first time was when he was 1 year old.

Billy is allergic to eggs.

Billy had these inoculations:

DPT-3 times-at 2 years old

BCG-1 time-at 9 months old

Polio-2 times-at 1 year old

Ask the nurse what other inoculations he should get.

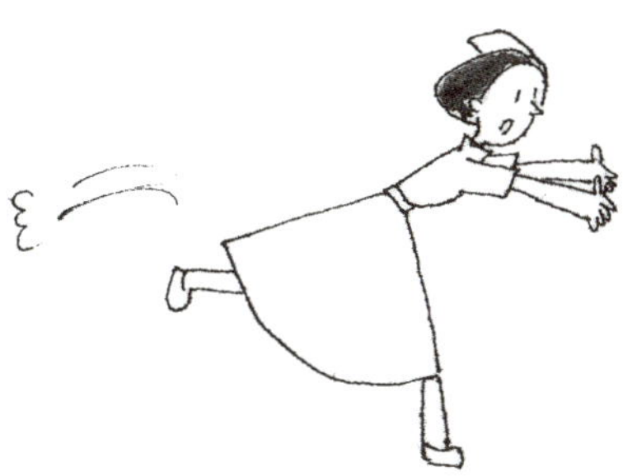

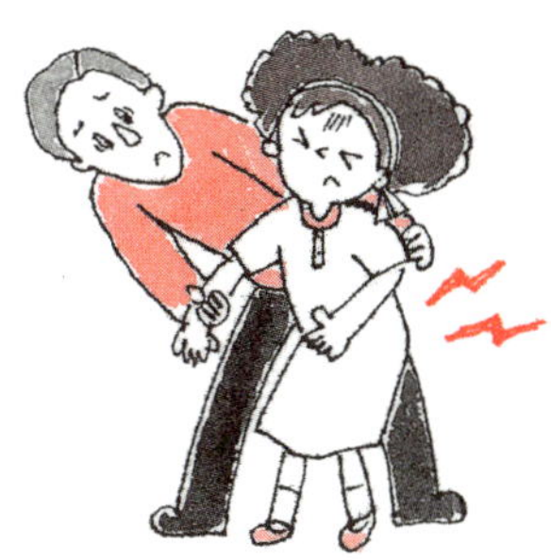

Activity 6: Game-Find someone Who

당신의 과거를 가르쳐 주세요.

교실내를 자유롭게 돌아다니며 클라스메이트에게 영어로 질문하여, 어린시절에 다음과 같은 경험을 한 사람을 찾아 보세요. 해당자의 이름을 기입하고, 다시 관련되는 질문을 당신이 생각하여 물어보세요. 같은 상대방에게 할 수 있는 질문은 3개까지입니다. 빨리 모든 항목을 채운 사람이 이깁니다.

예) "Did you fly in an airplane?" "Yes." "Where did you go?" "I went to Hawaii."
"비행기를 탔었습니까?" "예" "어디에 갔었습니까?" "하와이에 갔었습니다."

When you were a child···

1. Could you play a musical instrument?
Name ______
Q ______
A ______

2. Did you fly in an airplane?
Name ______
Q ______
A ______

3. Did you live with your grandmother or grandfather?
Name ______
Q ______
A ______

4. Could you ride a unicycle?
Name ______
Q ______
A ______

5. Did you go to camp?
Name ______
Q ______
A ______

6. Did you study English?
Name ______
Q ______
A ______

7. Did you move several times?
Name ______
Q ______
A ______

8. Could you swim?
Name ______
Q ______
A ______

9. Did you go to an amusement park?
Name ______
Q ______
A ______

10. Did you believe in Santa Claus?
Name ______
Q ______
A ______

UNIT 8

Your surgery will be tomorrow at 10 am.

한글 번역판 참조(147P)

Activity 1: Listening Practice

CD 23

Listen to the conversations and choose the correct answers.

1. How long does Mr. Edwards have to stay in the hospital after his surgery?
   a) one week b) three weeks c) two weeks

2. What kind of surgery does Ms. Smith need?
   a) pancreas surgery b) hernia surgery c) gallbladder surgery

3. What kind of anesthesia will they use for Mr. Horowitz's operation?
   a) general anesthesia b) local anesthesia c) epidural anesthesia

4. Where can Ms. Cotto buy the things she needs?
   a) at a convenience store b) at the hospital shop c) at a department store

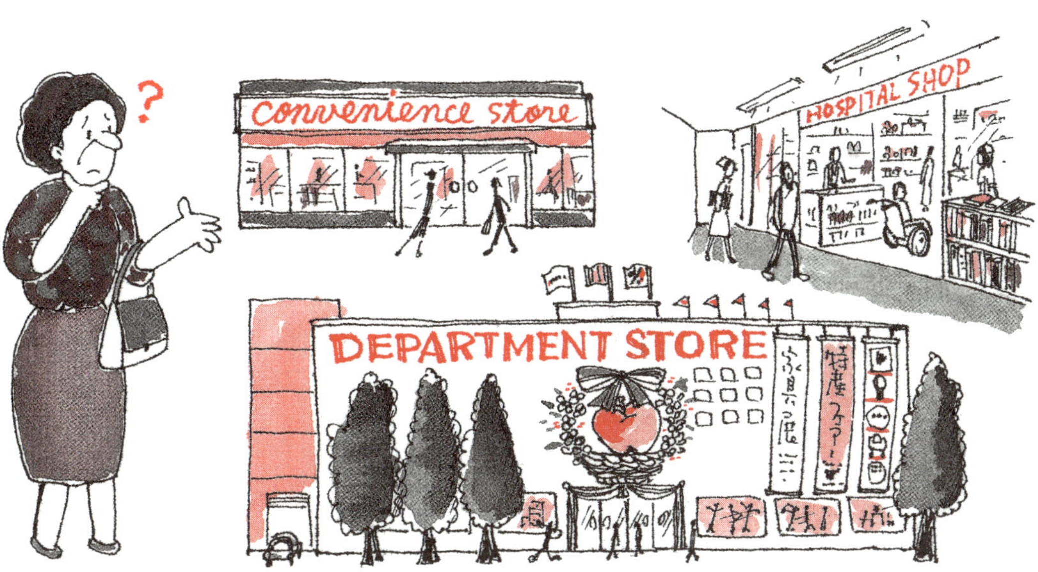

Activity 2: Checkpoint 1

CD

수술 전

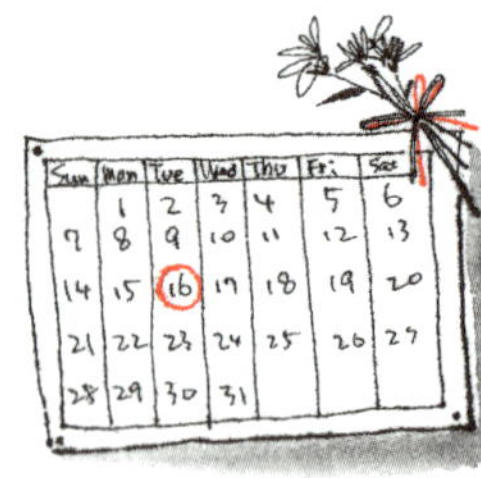

1. 저는 어떤 수술을 받아야 합니까?

What kind of surgery do I need?

당신은 장 수술을 받아야 합니다.

You need to have intestinal surgery.

2. 그들은 어떤 종류의 마취시술을 시행할 예정입니까?

What kind of anesthesia will they use?

그들은 전신(국소, 경막외, 척추) 마취시술을 시행 할 것입니다.

They'll use general(local, epidural, spinal) anesthesia.

3. 제 수술이 언제죠?

When is my surgery?

화요일 오후입니다.

Your surgery will be on Tuesday in the afternoon.

4. 제가 받게 될 수술에 대해 걱정이 됩니다.

I'm worried about my surgery.

걱정 마세요. 당신이 받게 될 수술은 아주 간단한 수술입니다.

Don't worry. Your surgery is quite simple.

당신의 주치의는 전문가입니다.

Your doctor is an expert.

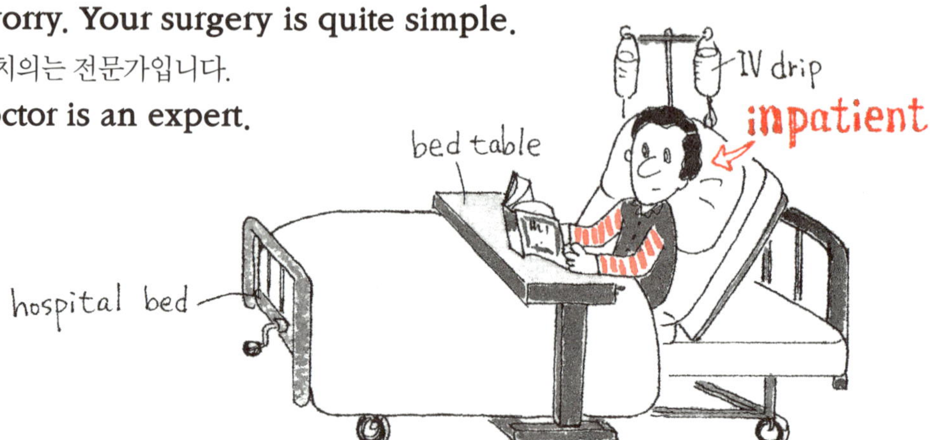

Checkpoint 2

CD 25

● 환자에 대한 설명

◇ 준비물품

Here is a list of things you need for your operation.

당신이 수술 받기 위해 필요한 물품의 목록이 여기에 있습니다.

You can get these items in the hospital shop.

당신은 이러한 물품을 병원 매점에서 구입할 수 있습니다.

◇ 의사의 설명, 승낙서

Your doctor will explain your operation.

주치의가 당신의 받을 수술에 대해 설명할 것입니다.

Your anesthesiologist will talk to you about your anesthesia.

마취과 전문의가 당신이 받게 될 마취시술에 대해 설명할 것입니다.

You have to sign a consent form.

당신은 동의서에 서명해야 합니다.

◇ 수술전날

I have to shave your abdomen*(chest, pubic area)*.

저는 당신의 복부(흉부, 음부)를 면도해야 합니다.

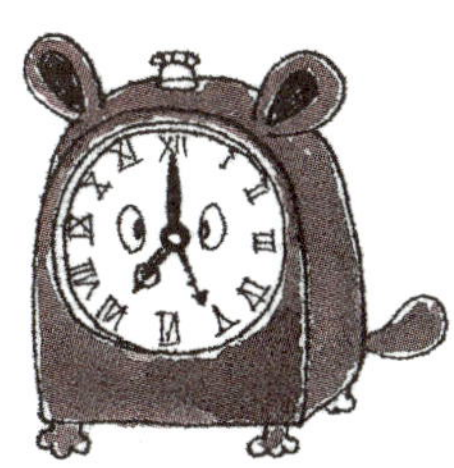

Please take a bath and shampoo your hair.

목욕하고 머리를 감으세요.

You will have a liquid meal.

당신은 유동식을 드시게 될 겁니다.

Don't eat or drink anything after 9 pm.

오후 9시 이후에는 아무것도 드시거나 마시지 마세요.

Please take this sleeping pill.

이 수면제를 드세요.

You have to wake up at 5 am.

오전 5시에 일어나야 합니다.

◇ 수술당일

I'm going to give you an enema; hold it in as long as possible.

관장을 하려고 합니다; 가능한 한 참으세요.

Please remove your dentures *(glasses, contacts, watch, jewelry)*.

의치(안경, 콘텍트 렌즈, 시계, 장신구)를 제거해 주세요.

Don't use any make-up *(hair product)*.

화장품(모발 영양제)를 사용하지 마세요.

I'm going to put a catheter in your bladder.

당신의 방광에 관을 삽입하려 합니다.

I'm going to insert a stomach *(gastric)* tube through your nose.

당신의 코를 통해 위관을 삽입하려고 합니다.

I'm going to start your IV drip.

정맥주사를 놓으려고 합니다.

We're going to give you your anesthesia.

당신에게 마취를 하려고 합니다.

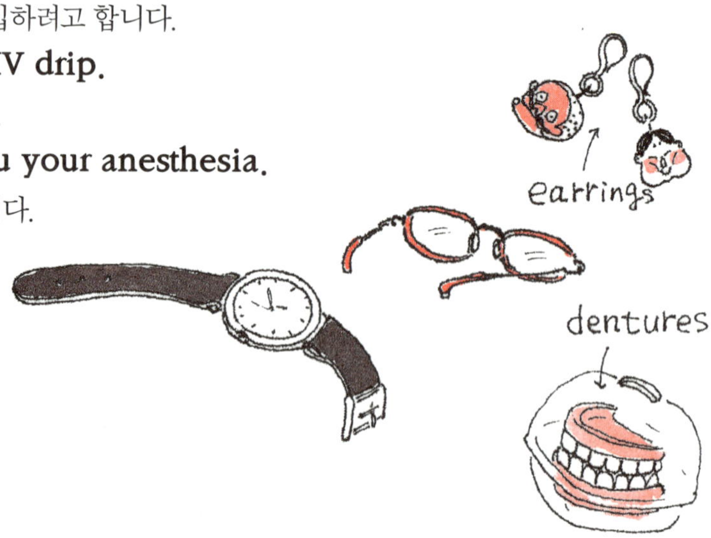

◇ 수술 후

We're going to remove your breathing tube.

호흡기 튜브를 제거하겠습니다.

We're going to bring you to the ward *(your room, the ICU, the post-op room)*.

당신을 병동(병실, 중환자실, 회복실)으로 모셔가겠습니다.

한글 번역판 참조(148P)

Activity 3: Dialog

CD 26

Listen to the dialog and fill in the missing words.

■ Two days Before Surgery

Hyoja: Mr. Brown, your stomach surgery will be on 1) ________________. There are some things you have to prepare for your surgery.

Mr. Brown: What do I need to prepare?

Hyoja: You need to have 2 paper 2) ____________________, 2 bath towels, 3 small towels, and your toothbrush and toothpaste. Besides that you have to have some special items for stomach surgery.

Mr. Brown: What special things do I need?

Hyoja: Here is a list. You can get these things in the hospital shop.

Mr. Brown: OK. I'll go there now.

Hyoja: After you get them, 3) _______________________ on everything in waterproof ink and put it all in the shopping bags.

■ The Day Before Surgery

Hyoja: Today is going to be a busy day for you. This afternoon the anesthesiologist is going to explain about your anesthesia. Then later 4) _______________________ about your operation.

Mr. Brown: I see.

Hyoja: This morning, a nurse will shave your abdomen. And after that you should 5) _______________________ and shampoo your hair.

Mr. Brown: OK.

Hyoja: Dinner will be your last meal; it will be a liquid meal. 6) __________ ____________________ or plain tea until midnight. At 9 pm, I'd like you to take this sleeping pill.

한글 번역판 참조(149P)

The Day of Surgery-Before Surgery

Hyoja: It's time to wake up, Mr. Brown. 7) ______________________; a nurse will give you an enema.

A Little Later

Hyoja: Mr. Brown, please 8) ______________________, glasses and dentures. Don't use any hair tonic. Please go to the bathroom, then change into this surgical gown and rest in your bed.

Mr. Brown: I changed into my gown.

Hyoja: Good. I'm going to insert a catheter in your bladder. Then I'm going to insert a stomach tube through your nose. Now, I'll start your IV drip. Just rest in your bed until someone comes to take you to the 9) ______________________.

In the Operating Room

Anesthesiologist: Good morning Mr. Brown. After you're asleep we're going to insert a breathing tube through your mouth. Now I want to give you an epidural anesthesia. Please 10) ______________________ and curve your spine as much as you can.

Mr. Brown: Like this?

Anesthesiologist: Yes, that's good. OK, all done. Now lie on your back.

After Surgery-In the Recovery Room

Dr. Yang: Mr. Brown, 11) ______________________.
Everything went well. You're in the recovery room now. As soon as the anesthesiologist says it's OK, we'll remove your breathing tube and bring you back to the recovery room.

Medical Terms - Surgery

Types of surgery

angioplasty	동맥 성형술
appendectomy	충수절제술
breast reconstruction	유방재건술
cesarean section	제왕절개술
cholecystectomy	담낭절개술
coronary artery bypass graft	관상동맥우회술
embolectomy	색전제거술
gastrectomy	위절제술
heart-valve replacement	심장판막 복원술
hemorrhoidectomy	치질절제술
hysterectomy	자궁절제술
lumpectomy	종괴절제술
mastectomy	유방절제술
organ transplants(kidney, pancreas, heart, lung, liver, bone marrow)	장기 이식(신장, 췌장, 심장, 폐, 간, 골수)
plastic surgery	성형 수술
pneumonectomy	폐절제술
prostatectomy	전립선절제술
splenectomy	비장절제술
tonsillectomy	편도절제술
vasectomy	정관절단술

Special Methods in Surgery

cryosurgery	냉동외과수술
laparoscopic surgery	복강경 수술
laser surgery	레이저 수술

Types of Anesthesia

epidural anesthesia	경막 외 마취
general anesthesia	전신 마취
local(regional) anesthesia	국소 마취
sedative	진정제
spinal anesthesia	척추 마취

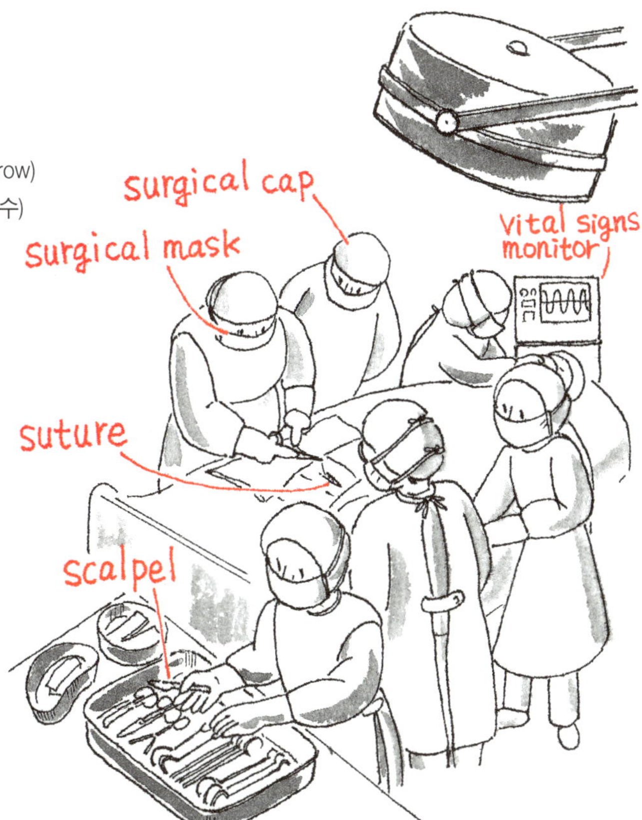

Activity 4: Puzzle-Body Parts

어느 부분일까요?

다음 표는 인체내부의 여러 가지 기관의 리스트입니다. 해당하는 번호를 그림 속에서 골라 괄호 안에 쓰시오.

( ) appendix	( ) gallbladder	( ) ovary	( ) small intestine	( ) tonsil
( ) bladder	( ) heart	( ) pancreas	( ) spleen	( ) ureter
( ) bone	( ) kidney	( ) penis	( ) stomach	( ) uterus
( ) brain	( ) large intestine	( ) prostate	( ) testicle	( ) uvula
( ) duodenum	( ) liver	( ) rectum	( ) throat	( ) vaginal
( ) esophagus	( ) lung	( ) rib	( ) thyroid	

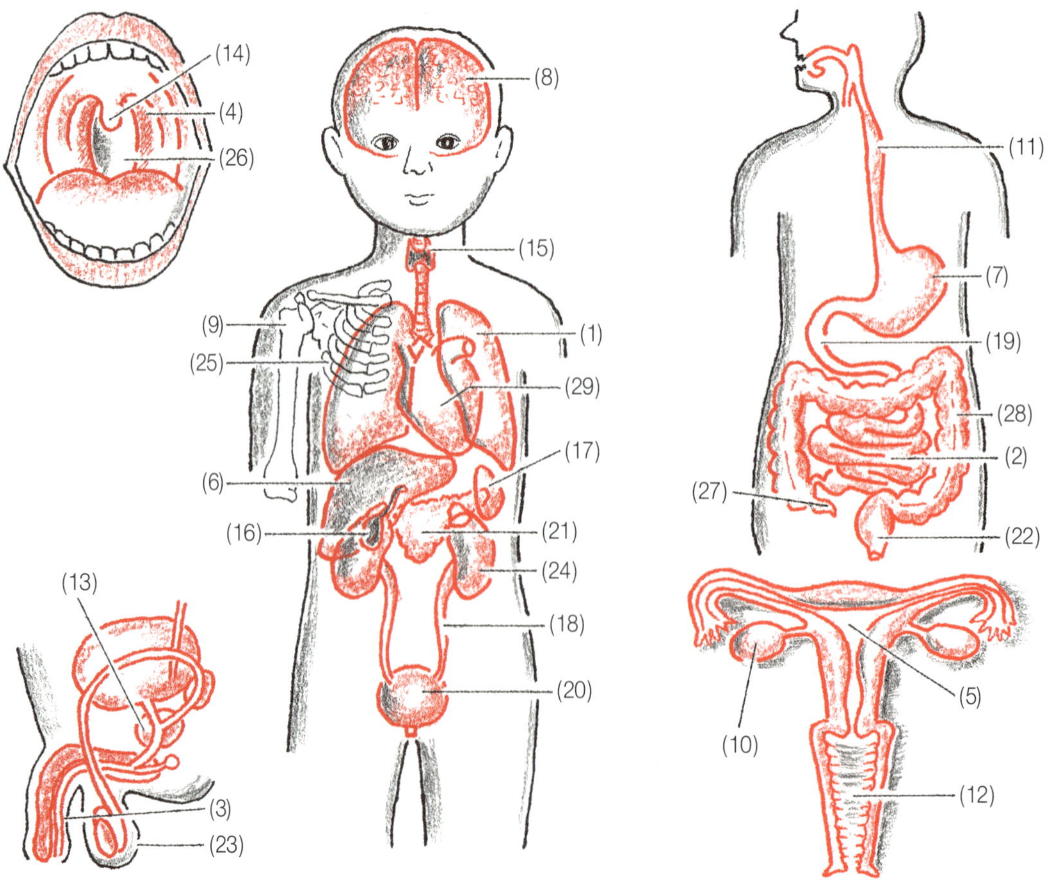

한글 번역판 참조(150P)

Activity 5: Role Play

수술 설명

2인 1조가 되어, 간호사역(A)과 환자역(C)을 정합니다. 간호사는 환자에게 수술에 관하여 자세하게 설명을 해 주십시오. 단어뿐 아니라 제대로 문장으로 이야기합니다. 환자로부터 질문이 있으면 그 질문에 대답하십시오.

환자는 간호사의 설명을 듣고, 카드에 해당하는 답에 표시를 하십시오. 간호사가 말하는 것을 모를 때는 서슴없이 질문하십시오. Checkpoint의 표현이나 Unit 1의 Emergency English를 참고로 하십시오.

끝나면 역할을 바꾸어, 이번에는 B와 C의 카드를 사용하여 연습합니다.

Role Card A-Nurse

Your patient is Barbara Jones. Explain about her surgery

Type of surgery: *Mastectomy(removal of breast)*

Day/time of surgery: *Thursday morning*

Type of anesthesia: *Sedative, general*

Length of stay in the hospital: *One month*

Items to prepare for surgery: *2 bath towels, 3 small towels, a toothbrush and toothpaste, 2 paper shopping bags, 1 gown, 1 cotton T-binder, 1 pare of underpants, 1 spouted water cup, 2 chest binders, 1 pair of pajamas.*

Day before surgery: *Adhesive tape test. Abdomen, chest and armpit shaved. Take a bath; shampoo hair. Sign consent form. Last meal will be a regular dinner. Take a sleeping pill.*

Morning of surgery: *Enema at 6 am. Remove contract, watch and jewelry. Don't wear make-up. Change into surgical gown and cap. Catheter and gastric tube will be inserted. Take a sedative.*

한글 번역판 참조(150P)

Role Card B-Nurse

Your patient's name is James Smith. Explain about his surgery.

Type of surgery: *Gastrectomy(stomach surgery)*

Day/time of surgery: *Tuesday afternoon*

Type of anesthesia: *Epidural, general*

Length of stay in the hospital: *5 weeks*

Items to prepare for surgery: *2 bath towels, 3 small towels, a toothbrush and toothpaste, 2 paper shopping bags, 2 gowns, 3 abdominal binders, 2 cotton T-binders, 1 pair of underpants, 2 spouted water cups.*

Day before surgery: *Adhesive tape test. Chest and abdomen shaved. Take a bath. Sign consent form. Last meal will be dinner, a liquid meal.*

Morning of surgery: *Enema at 7 am. Remove glasses, watch and dentures. Don't use hair tonic. Change into surgical gown. Catheter and gastric tube will be inserted. IV-drip will be started.*

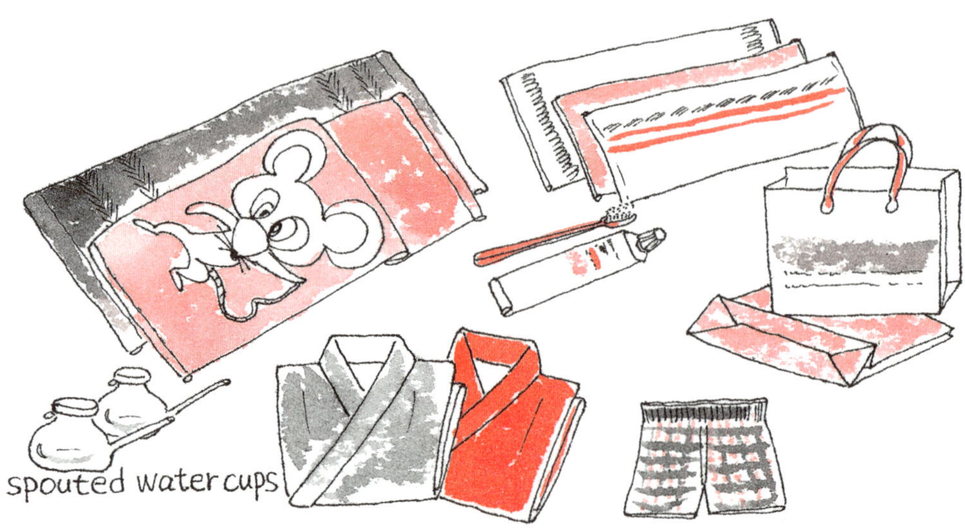

한글 번역판 참조(151P)

Role Card C-Patient

Listen to the nurse's instructions and check what he/she says. Ask the nurse questions if you can't understand or hear something.

Type of surgery

[ ]removal of gallbladder [ ]stomach surgery [ ]mastectomy
[ ]removal of pancreas [ ]intestinal surgery

Day/time of surgery

A[ ]Monday [ ]Tuesday [ ]Wednesday [ ]Thursday [ ]Friday
B[ ]morning [ ]afternoon

Type of anesthesia

[ ]sedative [ ]local [ ]epidural [ ]spinal [ ]general

Length of stay in the hospital

A[ ]one [ ]two [ ]three [ ]four [ ]five [ ]six
B[ ]day(s) [ ]week(s) [ ]month(s)

Items to prepare for surgery

[ ]towel [ ]toothpaste [ ]toothbrush [ ]shopping bags
[ ]gowns [ ]abdominal binder [ ]T-binder [ ]chest binder
[ ]underpants [ ]pajamas [ ]spouted water cup

Day before surgery

[ ]Adhesive tape test [ ]sign consent form [ ]take a bath
[ ]take a sleeping pill
Shave [ ]armpit [ ]abdomen [ ]chest [ ]pubic area [ ]neck area
Last meal A[ ]breakfast [ ]lunch [ ]dinner B[ ]regular [ ]liquid

Morning of surgery

[ ]enema [ ]bath [ ]change into surgical gown
Remove [ ]watch [ ]glasses [ ]contacts [ ]jewelry [ ]dentures
Don't use [ ]hair tonic [ ]make-up
Items will be inserted [ ]suppository [ ]gastric tube [ ]catheter
[ ]IV drip

Activity 6: Game-Pin the Organ on the Body

내 마음을 돌려 줘

이것은 눈을 가린 후 얼굴 윤곽만 그린 종이 위에 눈썹, 눈, 코, 귀, 입을 그린 종이를 얹어 완성하는 놀이형식의 게임입니다. 우선 큰 인체도(내부 기관이 몇 가지 빠져 있는 것)를 벽에 붙입니다. 누군가 한 사람에게 심장 등 기관의 그림카드를 하나 건네 주고, 눈을 가린 후에 빙글빙글 돌립니다. 그 사람은 스스로 인체도 있는 곳까지 가서, 기관의 그림카드를 그림의 바른 위치에 붙여야 합니다. 다른 사람은 영어로 다음과 같은 지시를 하며, 위치를 가르쳐 주세요.

예) Go forward/Turn around/Go left(right)/Turn left(right)/
앞으로 가세요./돌아 오세요./왼쪽(오른쪽)으로 가세요./왼쪽(오른쪽)으로 돌아가세요./

Move your hand(a little) up(down, left, right)
당신의 손을(약간) 위로(아래로, 왼쪽으로, 오른쪽으로) 옮기세요.

기관의 그림을 모두 붙이면 텍스트에 있는 인체도와 비교하여, 얼마나 정확하게 붙였는가 검사해 봅시다.

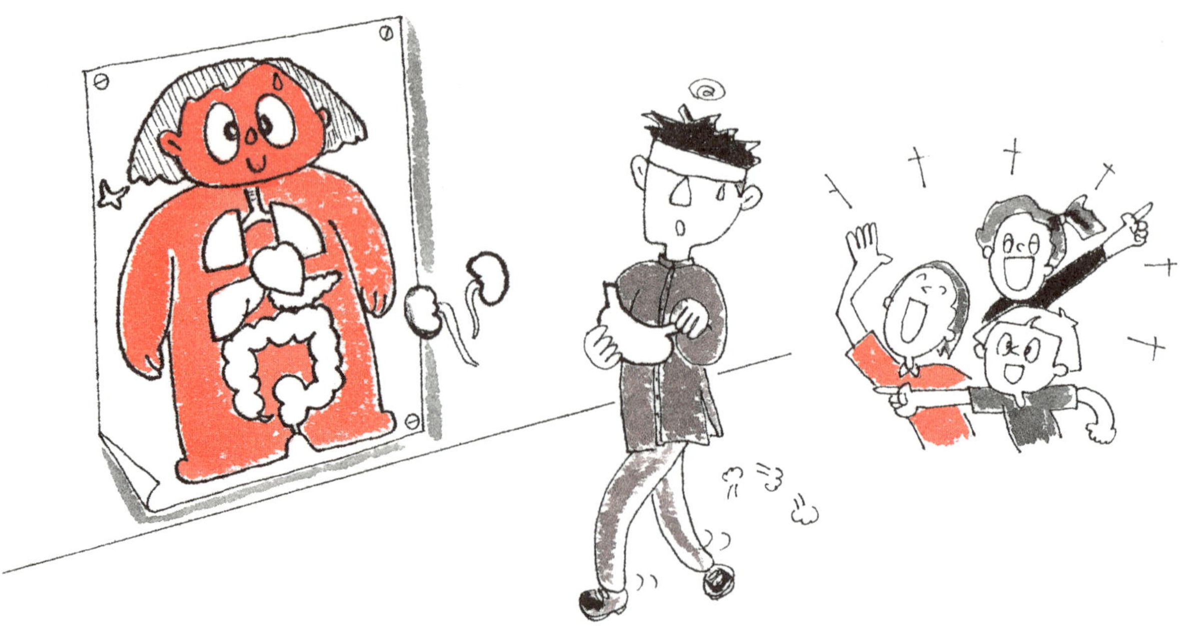

UNIT 9

How are you feeling?

한글 번역판 참조(152P)

Activity 1: Listening Practice

CD 27

Listen to the conversations and choose the correct answers.

1. What's Mr. Jones' problem?
   a) He has a backache. b) He has gas.
   c) He is nauseous. d) He has a fever.

2. How much of her meals did Ms. Appleby eat yesterday?
   a) She ate 30%. b) She ate 50%.
   c) She ate 75%. D) She ate 100%.

3. How many times did Maribel urinate?
   a) 6 times b) number 1
   c) 3 times d) number 2

4. How often should Ms. Silverstein take her medication?
   a) 130 over 84 b) 3 times a day before meals
   c) 2 yellow tablets and 1 pink capsule d) 3 times a day after meals

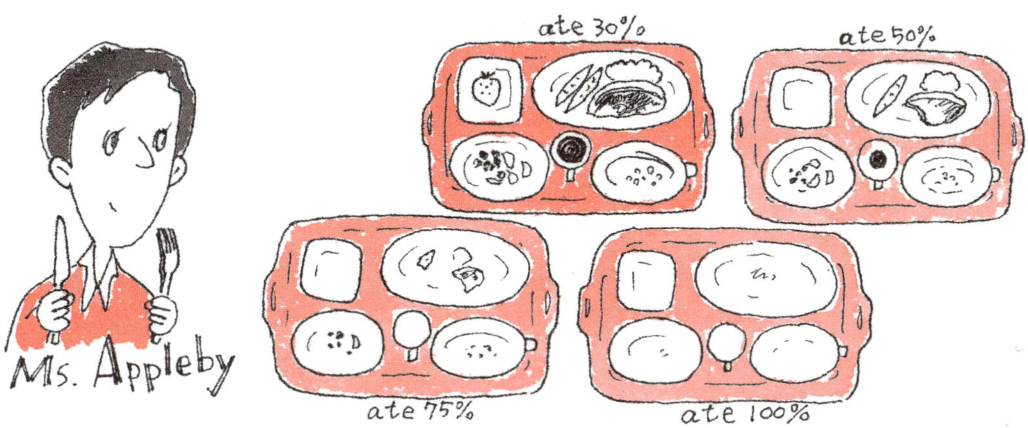

Activity 2: Checkpoint

CD 23

수술후/일상간호

1. 기분이 어떠십니까?

How are you feeling?

2. 통증을 느끼십니까?

Do you feel any pain?

3. 어디에 통증이 있습니까?

Where is the pain?

   허리가 아픕니다.

   I have pain in my back.

   수술부위가 많이 아픕니다.

   The surgical site is very painful.

4. 통증이 어느정도 입니까?

How bad is the pain?

   아주 경미하게(약간 아픈, 아주 심하게 아픈) 아픕니다.

   It's very mild(a little bad, very severe).

   통증을 참을 수가 없습니다.

   I can't stand it.

5. 진통제를 늘리겠습니다.

We'll increase your painkiller.

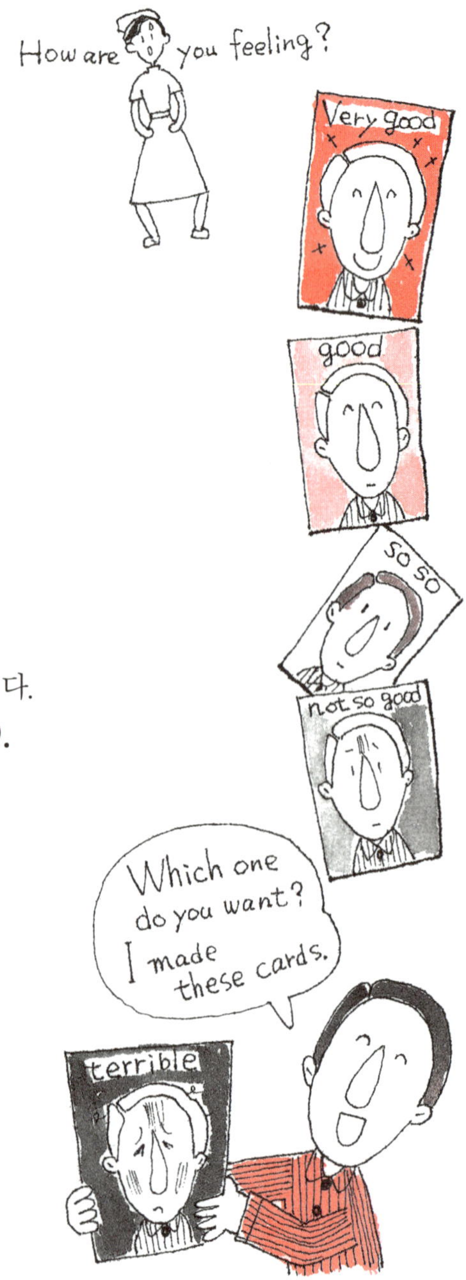
How are you feeling?
Very good
good
so so
not so good
Which one do you want? I made these cards.
terrible

6. 불편한 곳이 있습니까?

Are you feeling any discomfort?

머리가 아픕니다.

I have a headache.

오심이 있습니다.

I feel nauseous.

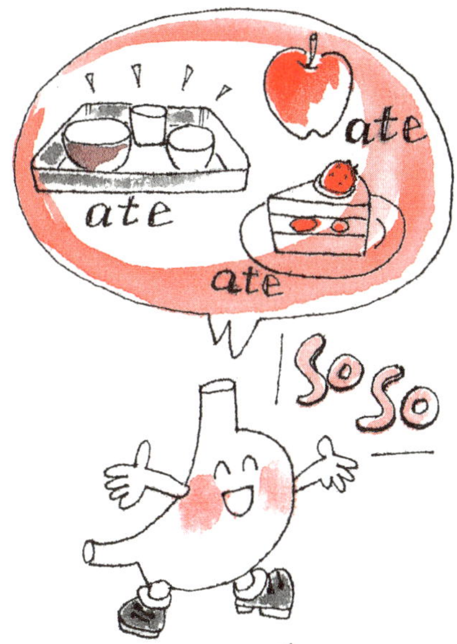

7. 식욕은 어떻습니까?

How is your appetite?

8. 식사량은 어느 정도를 드셨습니까?

How much of your meals did you eat?

식사량의 반(50%)을 먹었습니다.

I ate 1/2(50%) of my meals.

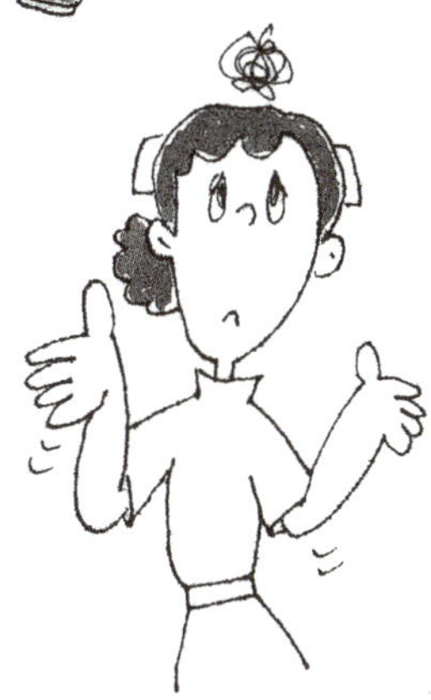

9. 혈압을 재어 보겠습니다.

Let me take your blood pressure.

당신의 혈압은 154에 85입니다.

Your blood pressure is 154 over 85.

10. 당신에게 주사를 놓으려고 합니다.

I'm going to give you a shot(an injection).

11. 당신에게 몇 가지 항생제(진통제)를 드리려고 합니다.

I'm going to give you some antibiotics(painkiller).

12. 어제 대변(소변)을 몇 번 보셨습니까?

How many times did you have a bowel movement(urinate) yesterday?

한 번(두 번, 여섯 번).

Once(Twice, 6 times).

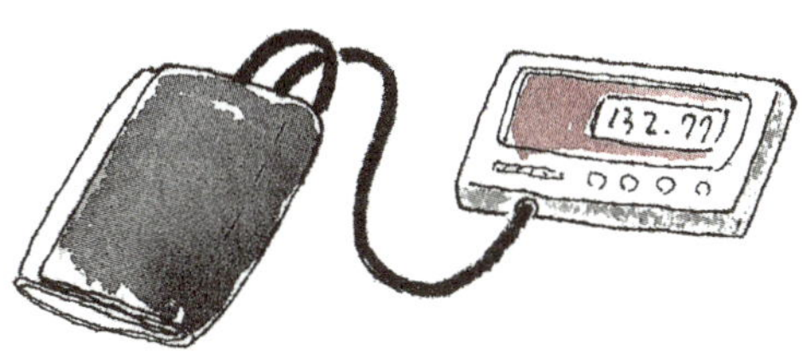

한글 번역판 참조(152P)

Note English–speaking people don't speak directly about urinating and having bowel movements. If they have to use the toilet, in America, they will ask, "Where's the restroom/bathroom/ladies' room/men's room/john?" In England, they ask, "Where's the WC/loo?"

Young children may not know the words "urinate" and "bowel movement" and those who know them might feel embarrassed using them. Most commonly, "Pee" "number 1" is used for urination and "number 2" is used for bowel movements. Adults might use ruder words like, "I have to pee/shit", but only among friends and certainly not in a hospital.

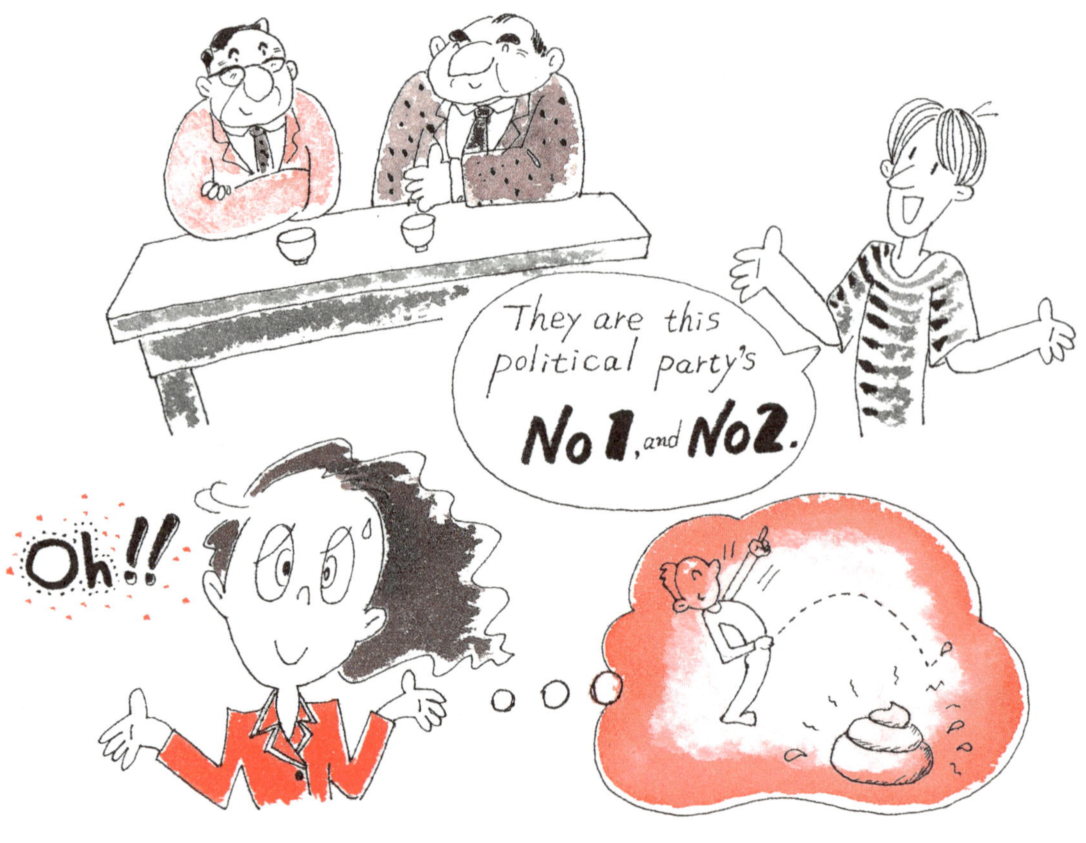
They are this political party's No 1, and No2.
Oh!!

한글 번역판 참조(153P)

Activity 3: Dialog

CD 29

Listen to the dialog and fill in the missing words.

■ Post-Op; In the Observation Room

Ms. Roberts: 1) ________________? Is my surgery over?

Hyoja: Your operation is over. You're in the observation room on your ward. You have to stay here until tomorrow. Are you feeling any pain?

Ms. Roberts: Yes, my right side hurts.

Hyoja: I'll give you a shot for the pain, but first I have to check 2) ________ ________________ and your blood pressure.
OK. Here's a painkiller: Try to get some sleep.

■ Later

Ms. Roberts: I feel very thirsty. Can 3) ________________ to drink?

Hyoja: Do you feel any nausea?

Ms. Roberts: Yes, a little.

Hyoja: Well, you can't drink anything yet, but you can 4) ________________ ________. That will make you feel better.

Ms. Roberts: OK.

■ Several Hours Later

Hyoja: How are you feeling?

Ms. Roberts: I feel better, but 5) ________________ .

Hyoja: Do you feel any nausea?

Ms. Roberts: No, not at all.

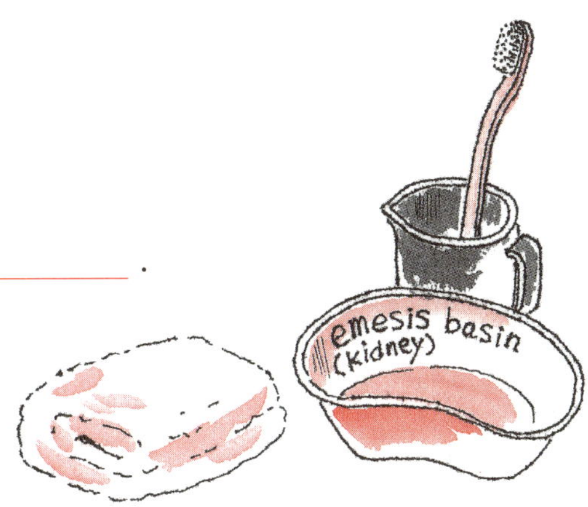

한글 번역판 참조(154P)

■ The Next Morning

Hyoja: Good morning, Ms. Roberts. How are you this morning?

Ms. Roberts: I'm 6) ____________________.

Hyoja: Your recovery is going very well. 7) ________________ remove your catheter and then you can be moved to your own room.

■ In Ms. Roberts Room

Ms. Roberts: Can I get out of bed today?

Hyoja: Yes, the sooner you start moving, the sooner your wound will heal. But you 8) __________________ the first time, so please ask a nurse to help you.

Ms. Roberts: I have to go to the bathroom.

Hyoja: OK. Please 9) ______________ and put your feet over the side of your bed. Stand up slowly and hold onto my arm.

■ The next day

Hyoja: Everyone, please return 10) __________________. The doctors are making their morning rounds.

Dr. Minjun: Nurse, please uncover Ms. Roberts' wound. Ms. Roberts, you are healing well. We can probably remove your stitches 11) ____________________.

■ Two Days Later

Hyoja: Good morning, Ms. Roberts. Here is 12) ___________________. Please take 2 capsules, 3 times a day after meals.

한글 번역판 참조(155P)

Activity 4: Puzzle-Scrambled Words-Matching

무엇을 하고 있는 곳?

뿔뿔이 흩어진 단어를 나열하여 바른 문장을 만들어 보세요. 또 각 문장은 다음 페이지의 A~P의 어느 그림에 해당할까요? 1)~16)의 번호를 기입하세요.

1) drip, finished, your, is ______
2) blood, I'm, take, going, sample, to, a ______
3) insert, into, going, I'm, suppository, anus, to, a, your ______
4) change, surgical, into, Please, gown, this ______
5) temperature, Please, your, take ______
6) is, your, pressure, 150, blood, 85, over ______
7) give, going, you, enema, I'm, an, to ______
8) need, bedpan, use, do, to, the, you ______
9) an, to, I, injection, need, you, give ______
10) dressing, have, on, change, your, the, to, wound, I ______
11) tomorrow, remove, the, will, doctor, stitches, your ______
12) first, the, take, to, elevator, floor, the ______
13) sample, cup, in, please, a urine, this, put ______
14) listen, I, to, your, want, to, lungs ______
15) feel, do, nauseous, you ______
16) call, toilet, a, to, need, please, if, you, the, to, go, nurse ______

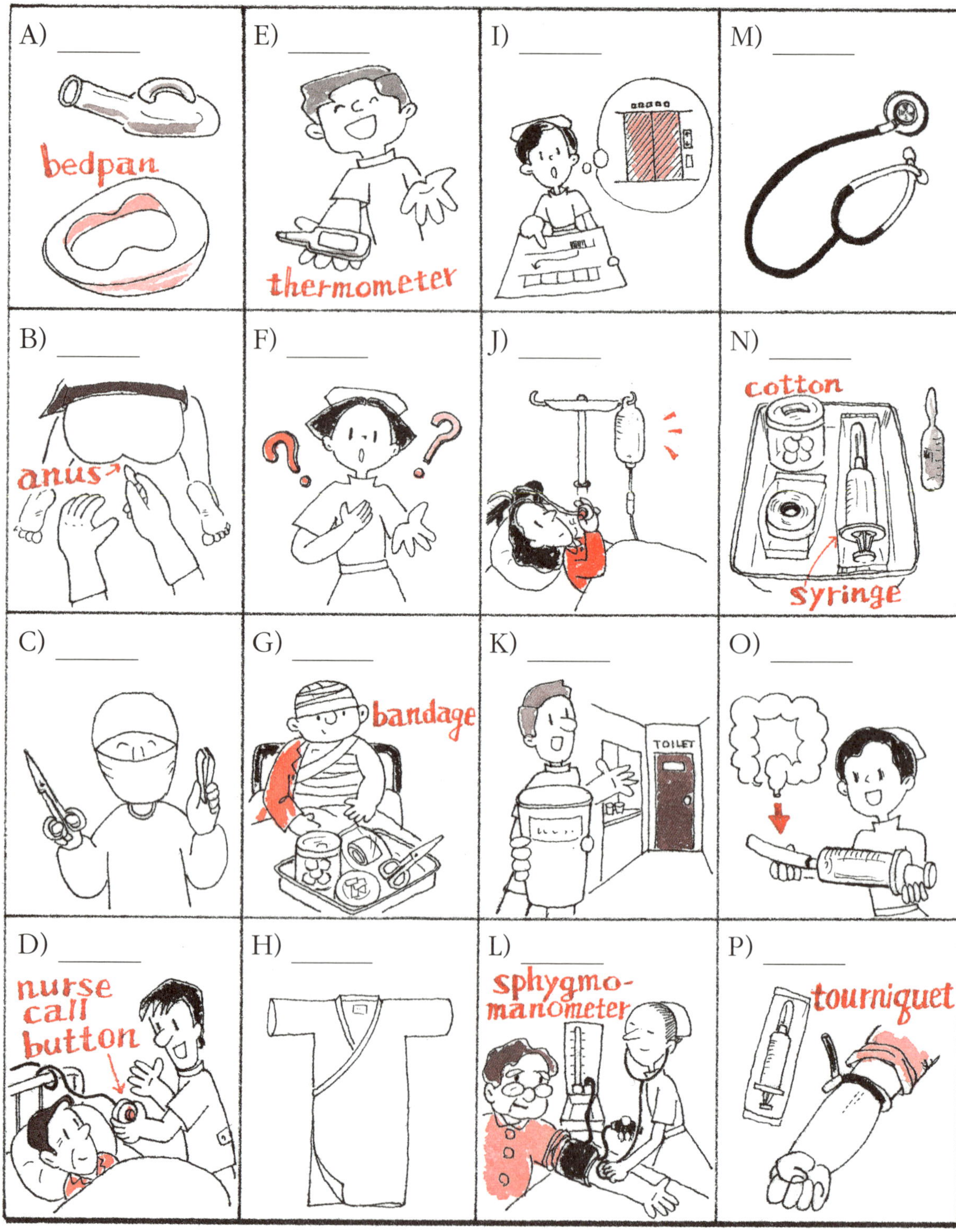
A) ______
bedpan
E) ______
thermometer
I) ______
M) ______
B) ______
anus
F) ______
J) ______
N) ______
cotton
syringe
C) ______
G) ______
bandage
K) ______
TOILET
O) ______
D) ______
nurse call button
H) ______
L) ______
sphygmo-manometer
P) ______
tourniquet

Medical Terms - Medicine

Internal Use Medicine

capsule	캡슐
liquid	물약
pill	알약
powder	가루약
syrup	시럽
tablet	알약(정)
throat lozenge(troche)	(목의 살균·소염을 위한)정제, (트로키제)

External Use Medicine

cream	크림
eye drops	점안액
inhalant	약 흡입제(inhaler 흡입기와 구분)
nose drops	코점적약
plaster	반창고
salve(ointment)	고약(연고)
spray	분무제
suppository	좌약
vaginal suppository	질좌약

How to Take Medicine

◇ 복용방법

Take 3 yellow pills, 2 red and white capsules, and 1 packet of powder, 3 times a day after meals. 노란 알약 세 알, 붉고 하얀 캡슐 2알, 가루약 한 봉을 하루에 세 번, 식후에 드세요.

Take this medication for 7 days. 이 약을 7일 동안 드세요.

◇ 삽입

Insert the suppository in your vagina(anus) every morning and evening.. 매일 아침과 저녁에 좌약을 질(항문)에 넣으세요.

◇ 바르기

Spread the cream lightly on your rash once a day. 하루에 한번 크림을 발진 위에 얇게 펴 바르세요.

◇ 사용하기

Use this inhaler twice a day. 흡입기를 하루에 두 번 하세요.

Take 4 puffs each time. 매 번 4 퍼프씩 하세요.

How Often to Take Medicine

Once a day, twice a day, 3 times a day, 4 times a day
하루에 한번, 하루 두 번, 하루 세 번, 하루 네 번

every 4 hours	4 시간 마다
after(before) every meal	식후(전)
after(before) breakfast(lunch, dinner)	아침(점심, 저녁) 식사 후(전)에
between meals	식사와 식사 사이(식간)
before going to sleep	취침 전
when necessary	필요시
as directed by your doctor	의사의 지시대로

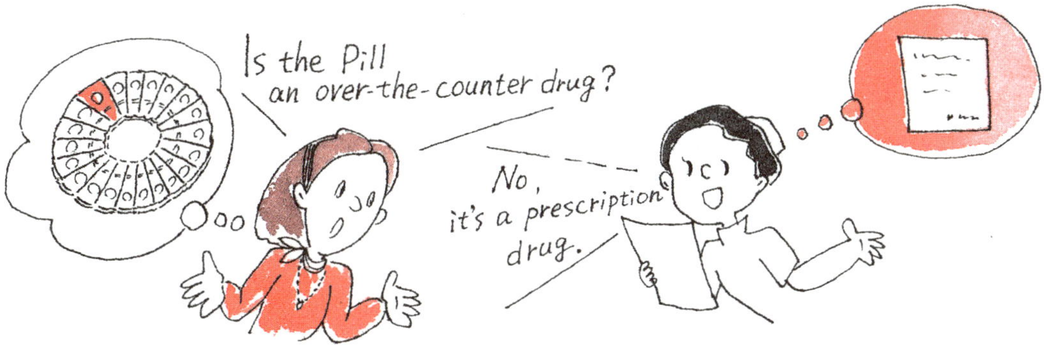
Is the Pill an over-the-counter drug?
No, it's a prescription drug.

한글 번역판 참조(156P)

Activity 5: Role Play

간호기록

2인 1조가 되어, 간호사역(A)과 환자(C)역을 정하십시오. 간호사는 환자에게 질문하고, 간호기록에 기입하세요. 끝나면 역할을 바꾸어, 이번에는 간호사(B)와 환자(C)의 카드를 사용하여 연습합니다.

Role Card A - Nurse

Your patient is Jerry Lopez. He had gallbladder surgery.

Ask him how he is feeling, whether he has any pain, about his appetite, his bowel movements and urination, and his temperature.

Tell him you're going to take his blood pressure. It's 150 over 95. Give Mr. Lopez his medication. He should take the white tablet once a day before going to sleep.

Write the information on the Daily Report Chart on the nest page.

Role Card B - Nurse

Your patient is Rosalie Galison. She had an abdominal hernia removed.

Ask her how she is feeling, whether she has any pain, about her appetitive, her bowel movements and urination, and her temperature.

Tell her you're going to take a blood sample. Give Ms. Galison her mediation. She should take 1 blue and white capsule 3 times a day after meals.

Write the information on the Daily Report Chart on the next page.

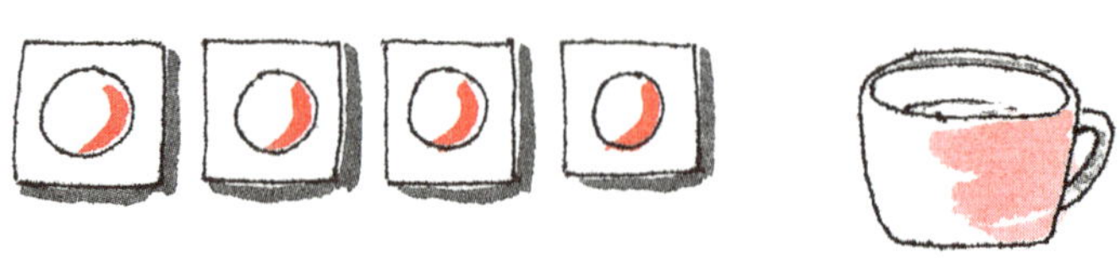

한글 번역판 참조(156P)

간호기록

환자명 ______________________

수술명 ______________________

주소 ______________________

통증 유/무 부위 ______________________

식욕 ______________________

배변 ________회 배뇨 ________회

체온 ________ 혈압 ________

처방내용 ______________________

Role Card C-Patient

You are Jerry Lopez. You had gallbladder surgery. You're not feeling very well; you couldn't sleep last night because you felt nauseous. You have a pain in your lower back. Your appetite is not so good; you only ate about 30% of your meals yesterday. You had no bowel movements and urinated 7 times. Your temperature is 37.9°.

Role Card D-Patient

You are Rosalie Galison. You had an abdominal hernia removed. You are feeling so-so. Your surgical site is very painful. Your appetite is so-so. You ate 60% of your meals. You had one bowel movement and urinated 6 times. Your temperature is 36.8°.

Activity 6: Game-What's the object?

무엇을 찾을까요?

이것은 그룹으로 하는 카르타게임입니다. 카드는 선생님께 받으십시오. 그림패는 겉을 위로 하여 책상에 펼치고, 읽은 패는 포개어 엎어 놓습니다. 누군가 한 사람이 읽어주고, 가장 위의 읽은 패를 집어서, 적혀 있는 영어단어를 읽습니다. 다른 사람들은 그 단어를 나타내는 그림패를 찾으세요(모두가 차례대로 읽는 술래가 되도록 합니다).

아무도 그림패를 잡지 못한 때는 적혀 있던 영어단어를 읽는 사람이 한국말로 설명하고, 그 읽은 패는 바닥의 패 속에 도로 넣어서 나중에 재도전합니다. 가장 많이 카드를 잡은 사람이 이깁니다.

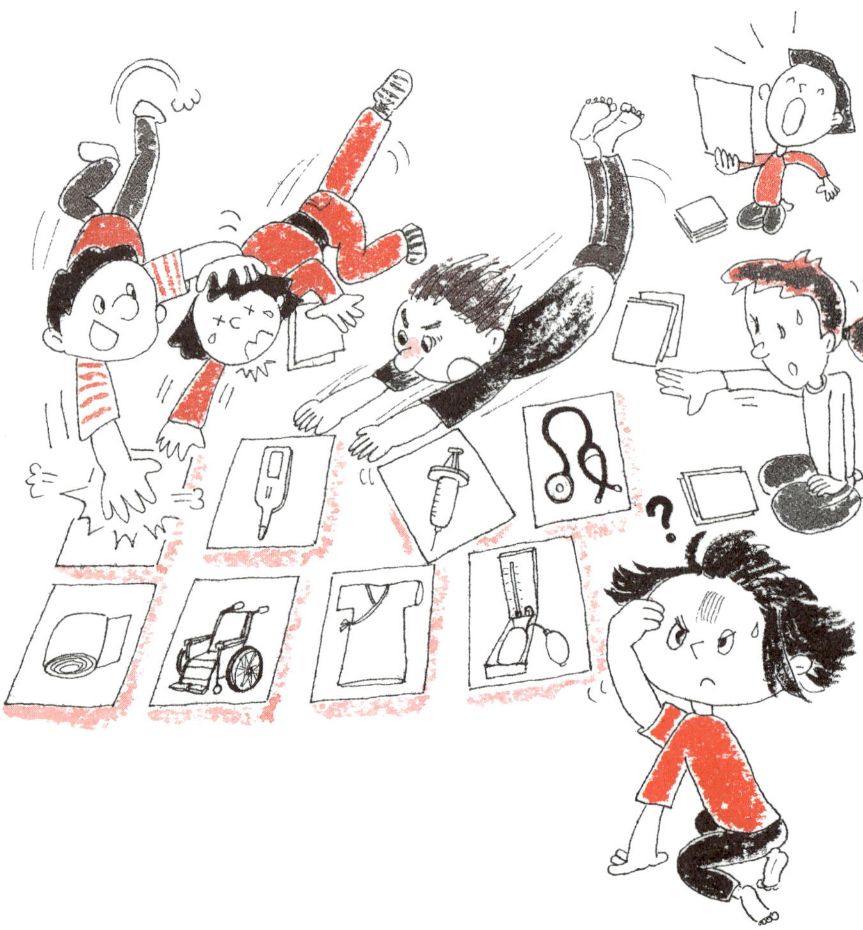

UNIT 10

Are you worried about anything?

한글 번역판 참조(157P)

Activity 1: Listening Practice

CD 30

Listen to the conversations and choose the correct answers.

1. What kind of foods can't Mrs. Lieberman eat?
   a) She can't eat cheese or pork.
   b) She can't eat any meat.
   c) She can't eat shellfish and pork.
   d) She can't eat any meals.

2. Why is Billy worried?
   a) He's worried because his stitches itch.
   b) He's worried because he's not healing well.
   c) He's worried because he's going to have an operation.
   d) He's worried it will hurt when the doctor takes out his stitches.

3. Why doesn't Mrs. Jennings want to have a blood transfusion?
   a) Because she's afraid of getting HIV.
   b) Because she doesn't want surgery.
   c) Because of her religion.
   d) Because she's worried about her surgery.

4. What does Mr. Philips want?
   a) He wants more painkillers.
   b) He wants to go home.
   c) He wants to talk to his doctor.
   d) He wants to stop taking morphine.

Activity 2: Checkpoint

CD 3

정신적 케어/문화나 종교의 차이

1. 걱정이나 근심이 있습니까?

Do you have any concerns or worries?

Are you worried about anything?

예, 제가 받을 수술에 대해 걱정이 됩니다.

Yes, I'm worried about my surgery.

정말로 수술을 해야만 합니까? 다른 의사의 의견도 들어보고 싶습니다.

I don't know if I really need my surgery. I'd like to have a second opinion.

2. 걱정이 된다면, 주치의와 상의해 보세요.

If you are worried, let's talk with your doctor.

제가 당신이 받게 될 치료법에 대해 주치의에게 물어보겠습니다.

I'll talk to(ask) your doctor about you treatment.

3. 당신의 종교는 무엇입니까?

What's your religion?

What religion are your?

저는 카톨릭(기독교, 이슬람교, 유대교, 불교, 힌두교, 여호와 증인)입니다.

I'm Catholic(protestant, Islamic, Jewish, Buddhist, Hindu, a Jehovah's Witness).

4. 당신은 종교 때문에 할 수 없는 어떤 제한 점이 있습니까?

Do you have any restrictions because of your religion?

저는 수혈을 받지 못합니다.

I can't have a blood transfusion.

5. 당신은 식사에 어떤 제한 사항이 있습니까?

Do you have any dietary restrictions?

저는 채식주의입니다.

I'm a vegetarian.

저는 돼지고기(소고기)를 먹지 못합니다.

I can't eat pork.

저는 코셔(율법에 맞는 음식)만 먹을 수 있습니다.

I can only eat kosher food.

6. 당신의 종교 때문에 꼭 지켜야 할 사항이 있습니까?

Do you have any requirements because of your religion?

음, 저는 유대인이기 때문에 제 아기가 남자 아이일 경우 포경수술을 받아야 합니다.

Well, I'm Jewish, so my baby has to be circumcised if it's a boy.

7. 한약을 포함해서 현재 복용하고 있는 약이 있습니까?

Are you taking any medications, including herbal medication?

한약을 먹고 있습니다.

I'm using Chinese medicine.

8. 현재 복용하고 있는 약을 보여 주세요.

Please show me any medications you are using.

9. 1인실을 원하십니까, 아니면 4인실을 원하십니까?

Would you like a private room or a 4-person room?

1인실을 원합니다.

I'd like to have a private room.

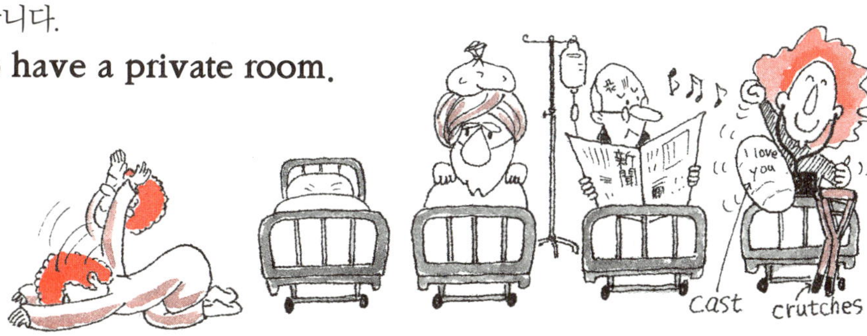

한글 번역판 참조(158P)

Activity 3: Dialog

CD 32

Listen to the dialog and fill in the missing words.

■ A Nurse is Visiting from America

Hyoja: Hello, I'm Hyoja Kim. 1) ______________________.

Carol: How do you do? My name is Carol Phillips.

Hyoja: Is this your 2) ____________ to Korea?

Carol: No, it isn't. I was an exchange student in Korea for a year in my university days.

■ Later

Hyoja: We sometimes have 3) ____________. Is there anything we should be careful about when caring for them?

Carol: In America, we have to treat patients of many different nationalities religions and cultural backgrounds. The most important thing is for doctors and nurses to realize that 4) ___________________________.

Hyoja: What are the most important differences?

Carol: We have to be careful about different peoples' attitudes towards doctors, hospitals and healing. For example, some ethnic groups, such as Koreans and Chinese, use herbal medications which may react adversely with the drug the doctor prescribes.

Hyoja: What are some 5) _____________ American patients?

Carol: I think 6) ________________ between Korean and Americans is that Americans want to know everything about their disease and treatment. They ask the doctor many questions.

Hyoja: Yes, I think that Korean patients are more passive.

Carol: 7) _______________ you have to consider is a person's religion. For example, if a person is Catholic they need to see a priest before they die.

한글 번역판 참조(159P)

Some religions don't permit blood transfusions. Also, some people have dietary restrictions. Islamic or Jewish people cannot eat pork. So it's important to find out about 8) ________________ and ask if he or she has any restrictions or special needs.

Hyoja: I didn't realize that religion is so important. Well, I'm glad I talked with you. By the way, there's an Englishman on my ward. I think 9) ________________ to talk with you.

■ On the Ward

Hyoja: Mr. Wilson, this is Carol Philips. She's a 10) ________________ America.

Mr. Wilson: How do you do? I'm pleased to meet you.

Carol: How are you Mr. Wilson? 11) ________________ being in a Korean hospital?

Mr. Wilson: Well, I'm really glad because Ms. Kim and my doctor can speak English.

Carol: Do you have any worries or concerns?

Mr. Wilson: To tell the truth, 12) ________________ my surgery. I'm wondering whether I really need it. In the west, we always get a second opinion, but in Korea it's not the custom.

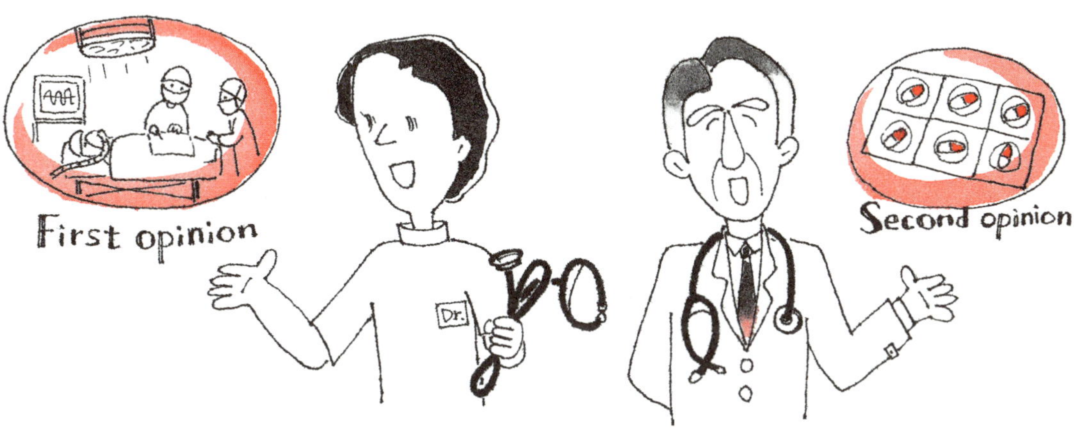

한글 번역판 참조(159P)

Carol: Yes, I can understand your concern. Perhaps, you should talk to your doctor again. Would you like me to be there when you talk to your doctor? Maybe 13) ________________ anything you don't understand.

Mr. Wilson: Yes, I'd like you to be there. My doctor said he'd come by at 8 o'clock this evening.

Carol: I'll be sure to come here before 8.

Mr. Wilson: Well, Ms. Philips, I was glad to have 14) ________________ with you.

In the Nurses' Lounge

Hyoja: I'm really glad that you spoke with Mr. Wilson. I 15) ________________ how worried he was.

Carol: I'm glad I was able to help.

Hyoja: I realize now that the best way is to ask the patient directly about his concerns or wishes.

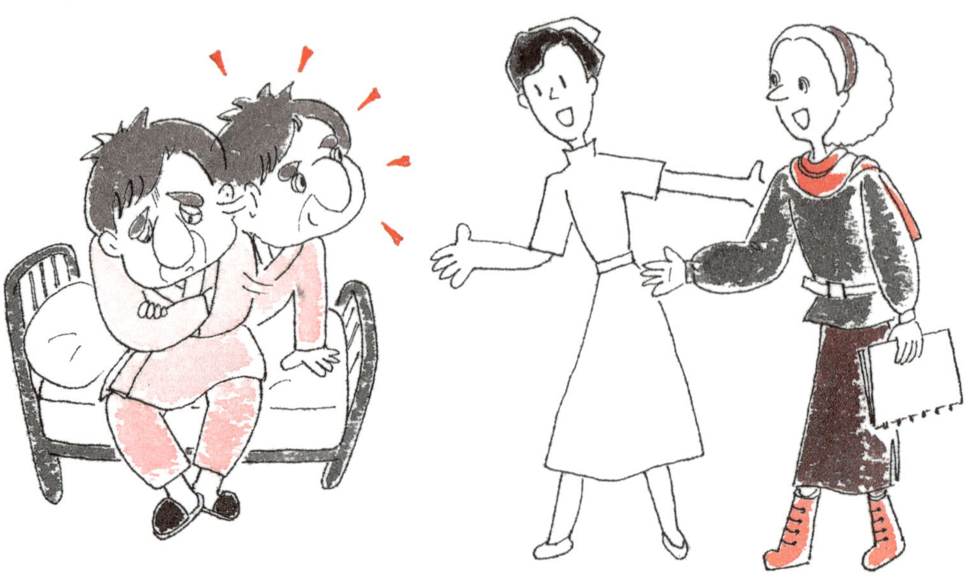

한글 번역판 참조(160P)

Activity 4: Puzzle-Quiz

각국의 문화와 종교

각국의 문화와 종교에 관하여 어느 정도 알고 있습니까? 당신의 지식을 체크해 봅시다. 단 해답이 한 개라고는 한정되지 않습니다.

1. Which is the oldest religion?
   a) Buddhism b) Judaism c) Hinduism
2. Which religion has the most followers?
   a) Buddhism b) Christianity c) Islam
3. Which groups of people use herbal medicine?
   a) Chinese b) Native Americans c) Koreans
4. Which religion prohibits the eating of beef?
   a) Judaism b) Muslim c) Hinduism
5. Which nationality believes that touching the head of a person may take away the person's spirit?
   a) Vietnamese b) Korean c) Polish
6. Which religion prohibits smoking tobacco and blood transfusions?
   a) Shintoism b) Jehovah's Witnesses c) Judaism
7. Which religion prohibits abortion and divorce?
   a) Judaism b) Catholicism c) Buddhism
8. Which religions forbid suicide?
   a) Buddhist b) Islam c) Catholicism
9. In which religion do boys become circumcised soon after birth?
   a) Christianity b) Buddhism c) Judaism
10. In which religion do women have to have a female doctor or midwife to deliver their baby?
    a) Buddhism b) Judaism c) Islam

한글 번역판 참조(161P)

Activity 5: Role Play

걱정거리에 대한 대응

2인 1조가 되어, 간호사역(A)과 환자역(B)을 정하십시오. 간호사는 환자에게 질문하고, 입원환자 면접표에 기입하십시오. 끝나면 역할을 바꾸어, 이번에는 간호사(B)와 환자(D)의 카드를 사용하여 연습합니다.

Role Card A - Nurse

Ask your patient questions to fill out the form.

Your patient is Muslim and can't eat pork.

He is worried that the insulin he needs for his disease is made from a pig's pancreas.

Tell him that you will explain his problem to his doctor and see if they can use insulin from sheep or oxen instead of pigs.

Role Card B - Nurse

Ask your patient questions to fill out the form.

Your patient is very old and can't walk by herself.

Tell your patient you will put a portable toilet next to her bed and a nurse will help her use the toilet.

Your patient is worried whether she really needs to have the surgery. Tell her you'll ask her doctor if there is some other way to treat her ulcer.

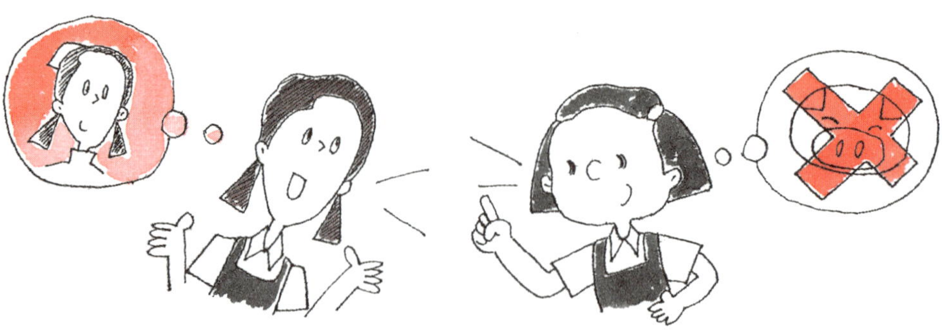

입원환자 면접표

성명 ______________ 연령 ______________ 성별 남/여

입원이유 ______________ 병실희망

국적 ______________ 종교 ______________ 독실/4인 병실

종교상의 제약 ______________

요망 · 특기사항 ______________

복용중인약 ______________

고민 · 걱정거리

____

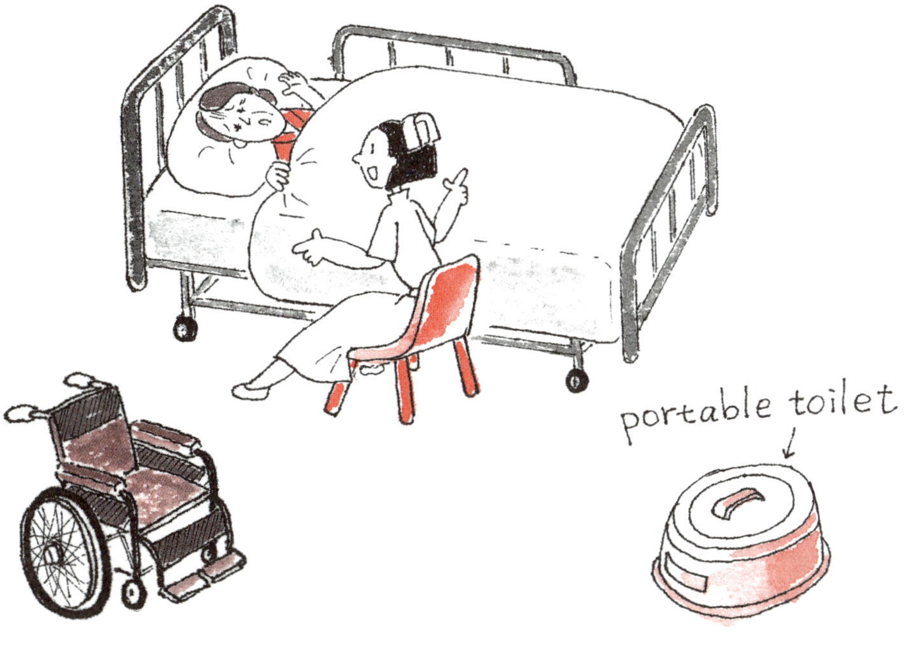

한글 번역판 참조(162P)

Role Card C-Patient; Abdul Mohammed, 46-year-old male

You were admitted because you have diabetes mellitus.

You are Egyptian and your religion is Islam. Your religion doesn't permit you to eat pork.

You'd like to say in a 4-person room.

You are taking medication for hypertension.

You are worried because you must have insulin to treat your diabetes and you heard that insulin is made from the pancreas of a pig. You can't take any part from a pig into your body.

Role Card D-Patient; Sun Wei Lin, 85-years-old female

You were admitted to have surgery for a gastric ulcer.

You are Chinese and your religion is Buddhism. You don't have any special restrictions because of your religion.

You can't walk by yourself, so you use a wheelchair.

You'd like to stay in a private room.

You are taking many kinds of Chinese medicine.

You are really scared of having surgery. You are very old, so you are wondering whether you should really have it.

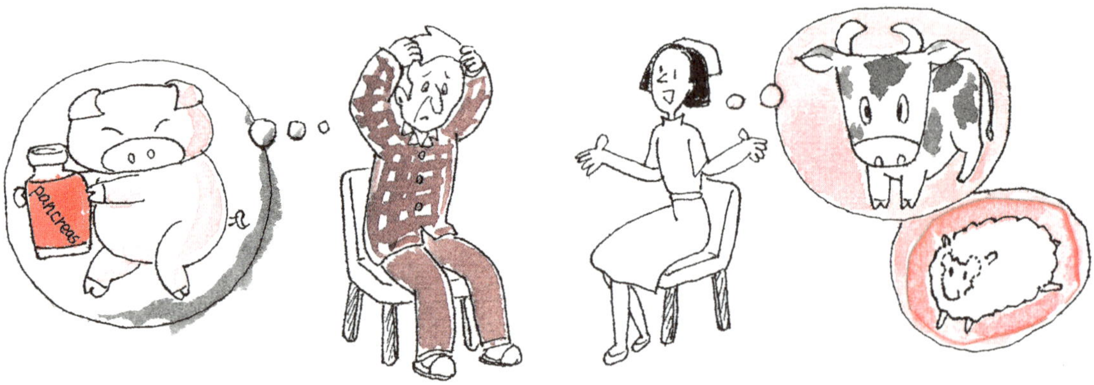

Activity 6: Game-What's the question?

무엇을 묻고 있는 것일까요?

그룹으로 나누고, 각자 말(지우개나 연필뚜껑 등)을 정하여 게임판의 START인 곳에 놓습니다. 부속 카드를 선생님께 받아서, 한 장씩 따로 떼어 잘 넘겨서 엎어 놓습니다.

한사람씩 순서대로 주사위나 동전을 던져서, 나온 수만큼 말을 진행시킵니다(동전인 경우는 겉이 나오면 1, 안이 나오면 2칸씩 나갑니다). 말이 멈춘 곳의 영문을 소리를 내어 읽고, 지시에 따라서 질문에 대답합니다.

TAKD A CARD라고 적혀 있는 곳에 멈춘 사람은 바닥에 있는 패를 한 장 잡고, 적혀 있는 영문을 소리내어 읽습니다. 다른 사람은 그 문장이 답이 되는 질문문장을 말해야 합니다. 가장 빠르게 골인한 사람이 이깁니다. 시간이 있으면 전원이 골인할 때까지 계속합니다.

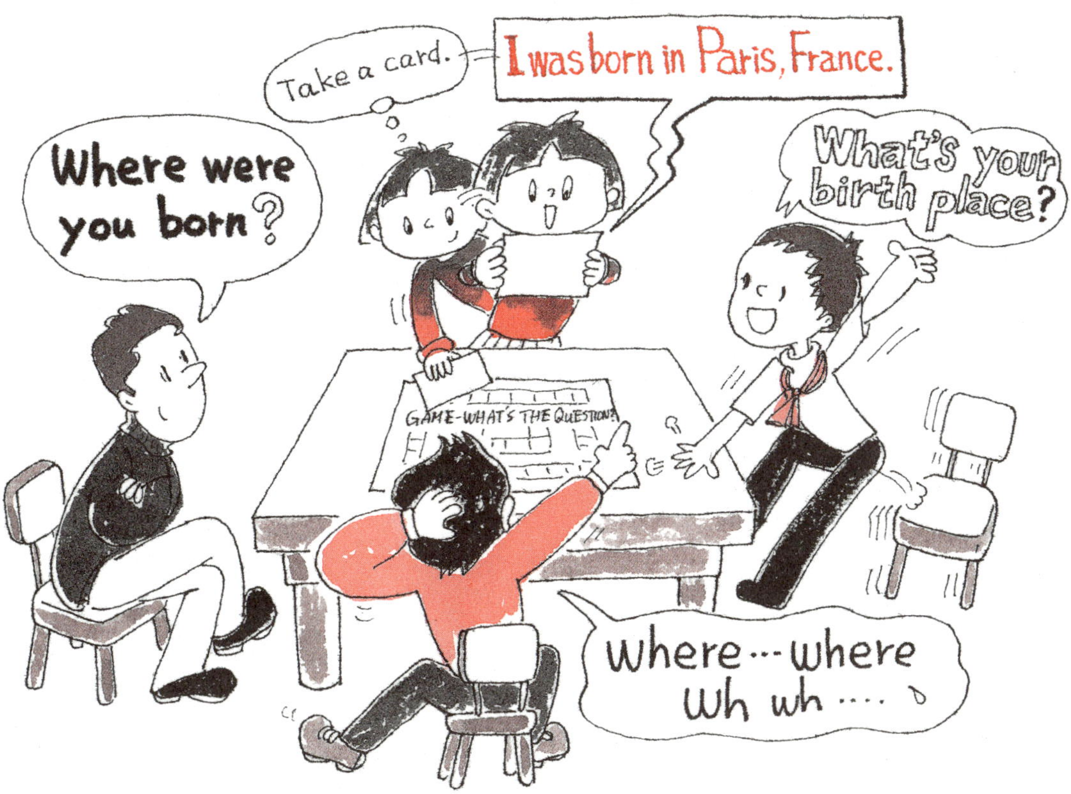
Take a card.
I was born in Paris, France.
Where were you born?
What's your birth place?
GAME-WHAT'S THE QUESTION?
Where … where
Wh wh ….

GAME-WHAT'S THE QUESTION?

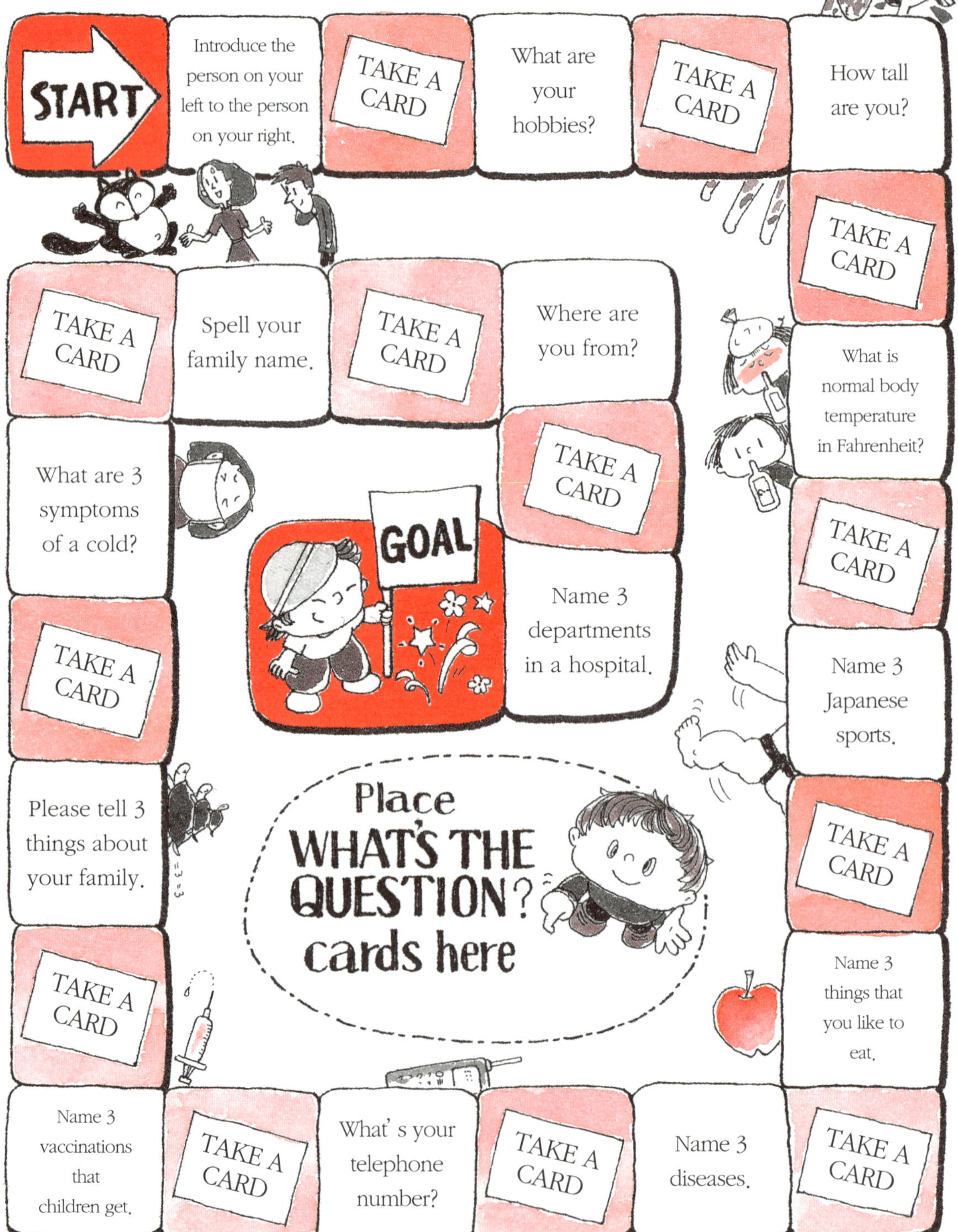
START
Introduce the person on your left to the person on your right.
TAKE A CARD
What are your hobbies?
TAKE A CARD
How tall are you?
TAKE A CARD
What is normal body temperature in Fahrenheit?
TAKE A CARD
Name 3 Japanese sports.
TAKE A CARD
Name 3 things that you like to eat.
TAKE A CARD
Name 3 diseases.
TAKE A CARD
What' s your telephone number?
TAKE A CARD
Name 3 vaccinations that children get.
TAKE A CARD
Please tell 3 things about your family.
TAKE A CARD
What are 3 symptoms of a cold?
TAKE A CARD
Spell your family name.
TAKE A CARD
Where are you from?
TAKE A CARD
Name 3 departments in a hospital.
GOAL
Place WHAT'S THE QUESTION? cards here

한글번역판

UNIT 1

당신은 외과 병동에서 근무하십니까?

1 페이지

연습1: 듣기 훈련

대화를 듣고 올바른 답을 고르세요.

1. 여자의 성은 무엇입니까?
   a) 들로레스
   b) 아르젠티나
   c) 아고스토
2. 남자의 전화번호는 무엇입니까?
   a) 02−6299−8614
   b) 02−6299−8641
   c) 02−6299−8614
3. 여자는 남자에게 무엇을 묻고 있습니까?
   a) 남자의 전화번호를 알고 싶어 합니다.
   b) 남자의 직업을 알고 싶어 합니다.
   c) 남자가 지금 무엇을 하고 있는지에 대해 알고 싶어 합니다.
4. 하비 존스씨의 직업은 무엇입니까?
   a) 산과 의사입니다.
   b) 간호사입니다.
   c) 의사입니다.

3 페이지

[초면인사]

1. [격식 차린 경우]

메리: 샘, 이분은 프랭크 쏘여씨입니다. 프랭크, 이분은 샘 헤르난데씨입니다.

샘: 처음 뵙겠습니다. 만나서 반갑습니다.

프랭크: 저 또한 만나서 반갑습니다.

2. [친숙한 경우]

메리: 샘, 이분은 프랭크씨입니다. 프랭크, 이분은 샘입니다.

샘: 안녕하세요, 만나서 반갑습니다.

프랭크: 저 또한 만나서 반갑습니다.

당신은 외과 병동에서 근무하십니까?

4 페이지

연습3: 대화

대화를 듣고 밑줄에 들어갈 말을 채우세요.

■ 효자의 첫날

수간호사: 앞으로 함께 일하게 될 사람 몇 명을 소개하려고 합니다. 효자, 이 분은 닥터 김민준입니다. 우리 병동의 선임 레지던트입니다. 닥터 김민준, 이 분은 앞으로 우리 병동에서 일하게 될 김효자입니다.

효자: 처음 뵙겠습니다, 닥터 민준. 만나서 반갑습니다.

닥터 김민준: 저 또한 만나서 반갑습니다. 잘 모르는 것은 주저말고 제게 물어보세요.

효자: 앞으로 도와주신다니 감사합니다. 또한 제가 일에 익숙해 질 때까지 잘 부탁드립니다.

닥터 김민준: 아. 저는 환자들을 살피러 회진을 마저 돌아야겠습니다.

수간호사: 4명의 간호조무사, 15명의 간호사와 6명의 의사들이 이 병동에서 일합니다. 또한 사무일을 보고 있는 사무원 한명이 있습니다. 나중에 소개시켜 드리지요. 간호사 휴게실로 가면 이제 막 교대근무를 마친 간호사들을 만날 수 있을 거에요.

■ 간호사 휴게실에서

수간호사: 이분은 김효자입니다. 여러분의 동료가 될 겁니다. 저는 할 일이 좀 있으니, 여러분 각자 효자씨에게 자기 소개를 해주세요.

효자: 저는 김효자입니다. 앞으로 이 병동에서 일하게 되었습니다. 여러분을 만나게 되어서 정말로 반갑습니다. 제가 처음이라 모르는 것이 많아 질문이 많겠지만 여러분께서 업무 요령을 잘 알려주시기를 부탁드립니다.

엘리: 효자, 저는 엘리 정입니다. 이 분들은 김지혜, 김인혜, 이도현, 정도희입니다. 물론 업무요령에 대해 잘 알려드릴 테니까 원하시는 것은 무엇이든 물어보세요.

효자: 감사합니다. 여러분 모두를 만나게 되어서 진심으로 반갑습니다. 여러분과 즐겁게 일할 확신이 들어요.

UNIT 1 당신은 외과 병동에서 근무하십니까?

5 페이지

도희: 우리도 새로운 동료를 만나게 되어 즐겁습니다.

엘리: 효자, 어디 출신이에요?

효자: 저는 완도입니다. 완도에 있는 적십자 병원에서 8년간 일했었습니다. 하지만 서울에 있는 간호대학을 졸업했고 그래서 다시 이곳에서 살기 원해서 왔습니다. 엘리는 어디 출신인가요?

엘리: 오, 저는 서울 태생이에요. 어느 간호대학을 졸업했나요?

효자: 국립 의료 센터 부속 간호대학 출신입니다.

엘리: 오, 저와 같은 대학을 나오셨군요. 제가 5년전에 졸업했으니까, 효자가 제 선배가 되겠군요. 지금은 어디 사세요?

효자: 병원근처에 아파트를 하나 얻었어요. 당신은요?

엘리: 저는 서울에서 부모님 그리고 남동생과 함께 살고 있어요. 효자의 취미는 뭐죠?

효자: 음, 테니스와 노래방에서 노래하는 것을 좋아해요

엘리: 저도 테니스 좋아해요. 언제 한번 우리 같이 테니스쳐요. 그리고 우리 모두 다 노래방에서 노래하는 것 좋아해요. 휴일에 노래방 한번 갑시다.

도현: 이번주 토요일에 일 끝나고 가는 거 어때요?

달, 지혜, 도희: 그거 아주 좋아요!

UNIT 1 당신은 외과 병동에서 근무하십니까?

8 페이지

역할 카드 A—간호사

당신의 환자는 한국어를 할 줄 모르는 외국인 입니다.
환자에게 다음과 같은 서류를 작성하기 위해 질문을 하십시오.

9 페이지

역할 카드 B—환자: 제랄드 브라운

아래 정보를 사용하여 간호사의 질문에 답하세요.

당신은 아일랜드 사람입니다. 1978년 10월 20일, 아일랜드, 드블린에서 태어났습니다. 당신은 여자친구 제니와 함께 살고 있습니다. 당신은 바텐더 겸 무용수 입니다. 주소는: 185—435, 서울시 강동구 성내동 522—11입니다. 집전화번호는 02—6407—4328이고, 직장 전화번호는 02—741—4494입니다. 취미는 조깅과 축구입니다.

역할 카드 C—환자: 메리 리 스미스

아래 정보를 사용하여 간호사의 질문에 답하세요.

당신은 미국인입니다. 1962년 8월 13일, 미국 뉴저지주, 트랜톤에서 태어났습니다. 당신은 결혼을 했으며 아이가 셋인데, 그 중 하나는 12살 된 딸과 10살 된 쌍둥이 아들이 있습니다. 당신은 치과 위생사입니다. 주소는 서울시 종로구 인의동 112-1 그레이스 맨션 407호입니다. 집전화번호는 02—561—7804, 직장전화번호는 02—471—4218입니다. 취미는 독서와 뜨개질입니다.

한글번역판

UNIT 2

어디가 아파서 병원에 오셨습니까?

11 페이지

연습 1: 듣기 훈련

대화를 듣고 올바른 답을 고르세요.

1. 그 환자분은 어디가 아픈가요?
   a) 그는 보험카드가 없습니다.
   b) 그는 허리가 아픕니다.
   c) 그는 정형외과 진료를 받기 합니다.
2. 제퍼슨 부인의 증상은 어떻습니까?
   a) 그녀는 변비가 있고, 기침과 열이 납니다.
   b) 그녀는 열과 기침이 나고, 설사를 합니다.
   c) 그녀는 설사를 하고, 요통과 치통이 있습니다.
3. 그 환자분은 무슨 과를 가야 합니까?
   a) 성형외과
   b) 외과
   c) 구강외과
4. 존스씨는 얼마 동안 위가 아팠습니까?
   a) 일주일 동안
   b) 이틀 동안
   c) 두 달 동안

14 페이지

주의: 한국에서, 체온은 겨드랑이에서 측정하는 반면, 서양에서는 보통 어른은 혀 밑에, 아기나 어린 아이들은 항문으로 측정합니다. 하지만, 최근에는 귀에 대고 고막에서 측정하는 빠른 귓속 체온계가 사용되고 있습니다. 이러한 체온계는 각각 체온계에 따라 정상 체온 수치가 약간씩 다릅니다. 대부분의 영어권 국가들은 여전히 섭씨보다는 화씨 단위를 쓰고 있습니다. 그들은 킬로그램, 센티미터 보다는 파운드, 피트, 인치 단위를 씁니다.

어디가 아파서 병원에 오셨습니까?

15 페이지

연습3: 대화

대화를 듣고 밑줄에 들어갈 말을 채우세요.

■ 외래 클리닉에서

효자: 버거론씨, 알렉산드라 버거론씨?

버거론: 예?

효자: 전에도 저희 병원에 내원하신 적이 있습니까?

버거론: 예, 있습니다. 2년 전에 내원했었습니다.

효자: 저희 병원의 ID 카드를 가지고 계십니까?

버거론: 예, 여기 있습니다.

효자: 이 서식을 작성해 주시겠습니까?

버거론: 죄송합니다. 저는 한국어를 읽을 줄 모릅니다.

효자: 알겠습니다. 제가 대신 작성하겠습니다. 그럼 제가 몇가지 여쭈어 보겠습니다. 당신의 성과 이름을 어떻게 쓰나요?

버거론: 알렉산더는 A-L-E-X-A-N-D-E-R이고, 버거론은 B-E-R-G-E-R-O-N 입니다.

효자: 감사합니다. 괜찮으시다면, 당신의 키와 몸무게를 알려 주시겠습니까?

버거론: 키는 175cm이고, 몸무게는 88kg입니다. 약간 과체중입니다.

효자: 나이도 말씀해 주시겠습니까?

버거론: 55세 입니다.

효자: 자, 오늘은 어디가 아파서 오셨습니까?

버거론: 숨이차고, 때때로 가슴이 조여 오면서 두근거리곤 했습니다.

효자: 이러한 증상이 있은지 얼마나 되었나요?

버거론: 이제 약 3, 4 주 정도 되었습니다.

효자: 가슴이 조여 오고 두근거리는 증상을 얼마나 자주 느끼셨나요?

어디가 아파서 병원에 오셨습니까?

16 페이지

버거론: 거의 매일, 특히나 계단을 오르거나 빨리 걷는 것과 같은 운동을 할 때 그렇습니다.
효자: 지금은 어디 불편하신 데가 있나요?
버거론: 아니오, 없습니다.
효자: 이 전에도 이렇게 심장과 관련된 다른 증상을 앓으신 적이 있습니까?
버거론: 아뇨, 없습니다.
효자: 전에 다른 질병을 앓으신 적이 있습니까?
버거론: 전에 이 병원에 입원하여 담낭 적출술을 받았습니다.
효자: 열이 있습니까?
버거론: 잘 모르겠습니다.
효자: 좋아요, 그럼 체온과 혈압을 측정하겠습니다.
곧 의사선생님을 만나게 되실겁니다.

19 페이지

연습4: 퍼즐—문장 맞추기

간호사: 열이 있습니까?
환자: 3일 동안 있었습니다.
간호사: 오늘은 어디가 아파서 오셨습니까?
간호사: 곧 의사 선생님을 만나게 되실 겁니다.
환자: 감기에 걸린 것 같아요
간호사: 이러한 증상이 얼마 동안 있었습니까?
환자: 예, 그렇습니다.
환자: 감기 증상과 두통이 있습니다.
간호사: 이번이 첫 방문 입니까?
환자: 예, 그렇습니다. 열이 38.2도 입니다.
간호사: 증상이 어떻습니까?

어디가 아파서 병원에 오셨습니까?

20 페이지

역할 카드 A—간호사

당신의 환자는 한국어를 할 줄 모르는 외국인입니다.
서식을 채우기 위해 당신의 환자에게 질문하세요.

21 페이지

역할 카드 B—환자: 알란 모스, 29살 남자

당신의 몸무게는 155파운드이며, 키는 5피트 11인치입니다. 당신은 어제 오후에 해변에서 발리볼을 하다가 발목을 삐었습니다. 발목이 굉장히 아프고 부었습니다. 당신은 정형외과 진료를 보기 원합니다.

역할 카드 C—환자: 산드라 필립, 52세 여자

당신의 몸무게는 138파운드이며, 키는 5피트 6인치입니다. 당신은 오른쪽 배가 아픕니다. 3일 동안 통증이 있고 매스꺼운 증상이 있었습니다. 어제는 두 번 구토하고, 열이 있었습니다. 열은 100도였습니다. 당신은 무슨과 진료를 받아야 할지 모릅니다. 간호사에게 물어보세요.

여기가 간호사실입니다.

23 페이지

연습1: 듣기 훈련

대화를 듣고 올바른 답을 고르세요.

1. 일요일에 방문객 방문시간이 어떻게 됩니까?
   a) 오후 2시부터 7시
   b) 12시 정각입니다.
   c) 11시부터 7시입니다.
2. 여자는 무슨 요일에 목욕을 할 수 있습니까?
   a) 화요일, 일요일, 월요일
   b) 월요일, 수요일, 토요일
   c) 화요일, 목요일, 토요일
3. 거동이 가능한 환자들을 어디서 식사를 할 수 있습니까?
   a) 레스토랑
   b) 환자 방
   c) 식당
4. 간호사 호출 버튼이 있는 세 곳이 어디 입니까?
   a) 식당, 환자의 침대, 간호사실
   b) 욕실, 간호사실, 화장실
   c) 화장실, 욕실, 환자의 침대

여기가 간호사실입니다.

26 페이지

연습3: 대화

대화를 듣고 밑줄에 들어갈 말을 채우세요.

■ 입원 교육

효자: 안녕하세요 마틴씨. 저는 담당 간호사인 김효자입니다.

마틴: 안녕하세요

효자: 담당 의사는 박준석 선생님입니다. 그리고 수간호사는 김호진 선생님입니다.

마틴: 알겠습니다.

효자: 옷은 여기 옷장에 넣을 수 있습니다. 나머지 짐은 침대 옆 테이블에 넣으세요. 이것이 간호사 호출 버튼입니다. 간호사의 도움이 필요하시면 이 버튼을 사용하세요. 짐을 정리 하신 뒤에 환자복으로 갈아입으시기 바랍니다.

■ 잠시 후,

효자: 오늘은 병동 오리엔테이션을 하려고 합니다. 저를 따라오세요.

마틴: 예

27 페이지

효자: 왼쪽이 간호사실입니다. 전화를 받으시려면 여기서 받으실 수 있습니다. 상담실은 간호사실 건너편에 있습니다.

마틴: 전화는 어디서 할 수 있나요?

효자: 병동 밖에 있는 휴게실에 공중전화가 있습니다. 화장실은 당신의 왼쪽에 있습니다. 소변검사를 하게 되면, 소변컵을 이 창문에 놓아주세요. 당신의 왼쪽에 있는 세면대에서 세수와 양치를 하실 수 있습니다.

마틴: 이 방은 무슨 방입니까?

효자: 이곳에서 세탁을 할 수 있습니다. 동전 세탁기와 건조기가 이곳에 있습니다. 세탁 이용시간은 오전 9시부터 오후 6시까지입니다. 식당은 당신의 왼쪽에 있습니다.

여기가 간호사실입니다.

28 페이지

식당은 302호 건너편에 있습니다.
검사실은 간호사실 옆, 왼쪽에 있습니다.
욕실은 화장실 왼쪽에 있습니다.
세탁실은 간호사실 건너편에 있습니다.
상담실은 간호사실 오른쪽에 있습니다.

29 페이지

병원에서 사용되는 물건

baby bottle 젖병
blood pressure gauge 혈압계
crutches 목발
emesis(kidney) basin 곡반
gauze 거즈
latex gloves 고무 장갑
microscope 현미경
oxygen 산소
sling 삼각건
stethoscope 청진기
syringe(needle) 주사(바늘)
vital signs monitor 활력측정계
X-ray 엑스레이

bedpan 변기
case 깁스
diaper 기저귀
examination table 검진 테이블
IV drip 정맥주사
medical chart 의무 기록
nurse call button 간호사 호출 버튼
scale 체중계
spouted water cup 주둥이가 있는 물병
stretcher 환자 운반차
thermometer 체온계
walker 보행기

여기가 간호사실입니다.

30 페이지

역할 카드 A—환자

간호사의 설명을 듣고 질문하십시오. 빈 칸을 채우세요.

당신의 간호사:

수간호사:

의사:

방문객 방문 시간:

31 페이지

역할 카드 B—간호사

당신에 대해 소개하고 환자에게 붉은색의 정보에 대해 설명하세요.

간호사: 당신의 이름

수간호사: 김호진

의사: 박준석

방문객 방문 시간: 오후 2시~오후 7시

역할 카드 C—간호사

당신에 대해 소개하고 붉은색의 정보에 대해 설명하세요.

간호사: 당신의 이름

수간호사: 강윤숙

의사: 김경운

방문객 방문 시간: 오후 1시~오후 8시

당신은 질환을 앓고 계십니까?

33 페이지

연습1: 듣기 훈련

대화를 듣고 올바른 답을 고르세요.

1. 김민준씨는 누구입니까?
   a) 그는 케인의 주치의입니다.
   b) 그는 케인의 아들입니다.
   c) 그는 케인의 남편입니다.
2. 케인씨는 어떤 식이제한을 하고 있습니까?
   a) 그녀는 쌀을 먹지 않습니다.
   b) 그녀는 매우 짠 음식을 먹지 않습니다.
   c) 그녀는 돼지고기를 먹지 않습니다.
3. 케인씨는 술을 마십니까?
   a) 아니오, 2년 전에 끊었습니다.
   b) 그녀는 매일 한 잔씩 마십니다.
   c) 그녀는 하루에 7잔씩 마십니다.
4. 케인씨의 아버지는 어떻게 돌아가셨습니까?
   a) 그는 심장마비로 돌아가셨습니다.
   b) 그는 고혈압으로 돌아가셨습니다.
   c) 그는 당뇨로 돌아가셨습니다.

당신은 질환을 앓고 계십니까?

36 페이지

연습3: 대화

대화를 듣고 밑줄에 들어갈 말을 채우세요.

■ 입원 인터뷰

효자: 한국에서 병원에 입원하신 적이 이번이 처음입니까?

케인: 예, 그렇습니다.

효자: 오늘은 무슨 일로 입원하셨습니까?

케인: 오른쪽에 통증이 있어서 왔습니다. 제 주치의 말에 의하면 아마도 충수돌기염 같다고 했습니다.

효자: 이 전에 심각한 질환을 앓아보신 적이 있습니까?

케인: 고혈압을 앓고 있습니다. 심장 질환도 있습니다. 그리고 3년 전에 교통사고를 당해서 걷지를 못합니다.

효자: 전염성 질환을 앓고 계십니까?

케인: 아니오. 없습니다.

효자: 수혈을 받아 보신 적이 있습니까?

케인: 아니오, 없습니다.

효자: 지금 드시고 있는 약이 있습니까?

케인: 예, 고혈압과 심장질환에 관계된 약물을 복용중입니다.

효자: 그 약을 제게 주시면 담당 주치의 선생님께 보여드리겠습니다.

케인: 알겠습니다.

한글번역판

UNIT 4

당신은 질환을 앓고 계십니까?

37 페이지

효자: 알러지가 있습니까?

케인: 예, 땅콩에 알러지가 있습니다.

효자: 약물에 대한 알러지가 있습니까?

케인: 아니오, 없습니다.

효자: 목욕이나 식사와 같은 일상생활을 하는데 도움이 필요하신가요?

케인: 음, 저는 휠체어를 잘 사용하기 때문에 목욕탕으로 들어가고 나올 때 정도만 도움이 필요합니다. 하지만 평상시 혼자 목욕하고 집에서 요리도 합니다.

효자: 시력과 청력은 어떻습니까?

케인: 시력, 청력 모두 좋습니다.

효자: 당신의 성격을 어떻게 표현하시겠습니까?

케인: 제 생각엔 밝고, 외향적인 것 같습니다.

효자: 종교에 대해 말씀해 주시겠습니까?

케인: 개신교입니다.

효자: 당신의 질병과 입원에 대해 걱정되거나 염려되는 점이 있습니까?

케인: 수술에 대해 걱정이 됩니다. 또한 제 주치의와 담당 간호사가 영어를 할 수 있는 분들인지에 대해도 염려됩니다.

효자: 걱정 마세요. 당신의 주치의는 영어를 할 수 있는 분입니다. 또한 몇몇 간호사는 영어를 할 수 있고, 또한 말씀하실 사항이 있으면 저한테 질문하셔도 됩니다.

4 당신은 질환을 앓고 계십니까?

41 페이지

역할 카드 A—간호사

당신은 입원 인터뷰를 하고 있습니다. 환자에게 그 혹은 그녀의 가족 구성도와 가족의 병력, 식이, 제한 식이, 흡연, 음주습관과 종교, 성격에 관한 질문을 하십시오. 다음 서류를 작성하십시오.

43 페이지

역할카드 B—환자: 노마 제임스, 39세 여자

당신은 유부녀입니다. 당신의 남편의 성함은 밥 제임스입니다. 그는 43세 입니다. 두 아이가 있는데 한 명은 8살 난 아들, 로드니이고, 다른 한 명은 12살 난 딸 메리입니다. 당신의 어머니와 아버지 모두 생존해 계십니다. 어머니는 2년 동안 알츠하이머병을 앓고 계십니다. 아버지는 3년 동안 당뇨를 앓고 있습니다. 당신은 건강한 남동생이 한 명 있습니다.

당신은 5살 이후로 천식을 앓고 있으며, 작년에 자궁암을 진단 받았습니다. 자궁적출술을 받아 지금은 괜찮습니다. 당신은 페니실린과 땅콩에 알러지가 있습니다.

당신은 하루에 세끼를 먹습니다. 당신은 유태인이기 때문에 돼지고기와 갑각류를 먹지 못합니다. 당신은 흡연을 하지 않으나, 거의 매일 와인이나 맥주 한 잔씩 마십니다.

당신의 성격은 외향적이며 명랑합니다.

역할카드 C—환자: 스티븐 엔더슨, 53세 남자

당신은 동성연애자입니다. 당신은 앤드류 필립이라는 파트너와 함께 삽니다. 그는 49세입니다. 당신의 어머니는 살아계시지만, 당신의 아버지는 4년 전에 뇌졸중으로 79세 나이에 돌아가셨습니다. 그는 오랫동안 심장질환을 앓고 있었습니다. 75세인 당신의 어머니는 4년 전에 담낭 제거술을 받았습니다. 당신은 두 명의 여동생이 있는데 한 명은 50세인 신씨아이고 다른 한 명은 48세인 엘렌입니다. 신씨아는 담낭질환을 앓고 있으며, 엘린은 건강합니다.

당신은 1997년에 HIV에 감염이 되었습니다. 두 달 동안 기침을 하였습니다. 당신은 먼지와 곰팡이, 꽃가루에 알러지가 있습니다.

당신은 채식주의자입니다. 그래서 고기나 생선류를 먹지 않습니다. 당신은 담배를 피지 않지만, 때때로 술은 마십니다. 당시는 개신교 신자입니다.

당신은 심각하고, 신경질적이며, 걱정이 많은 소심한 성격입니다.

UNIT 한글번역판

5 당신은 MRI검사를 받아야 합니다.

45 페이지

연습1: 듣기 훈련

대화를 듣고 올바른 답을 고르세요.

1. 간호사가 무엇을 하고 있습니까?
   a) 환자의 맥박을 측정하고 있다.
   b) 혈액을 채취하고 있다.
   c) 혈압을 측정하고 있다.
   d) 시력 검사를 하고 있다.
2. 실버씨는 언제 검사를 받아야 합니까?
   a) 수술 동안
   b) 오늘
   c) 수술 후에
   d) 입원 후에
3. 의사는 잭슨씨의 어느 신체부위를 검사하기를 원합니까?
   a) 구강
   b) 위
   c) 심장
   d) 대장
4. 김씨는 무슨 검사를 받아야 합니까?
   a) 방사선 동위원소 검사
   b) 엑스레이 검사
   c) 뇌파 검사
   d) MRI 검사

당신은 MRI검사를 받아야 합니다.

48 페이지

연습3: 대화

대화를 듣고 밑줄에 들어갈 말을 채우세요.

■ 병원에서 하는 검사

효자: 미스 양, 당신은 이번 주에 몇 가지 검사를 받으셔야 합니다.

미스 양: 무슨 검사를 받아야 하나요?

효자: 흉부 엑스레이, 심전도, 위내시경과 상부, 하부 소화기계 조영검사를 받아야 합니다.

미스 양: 흉부 엑스레이와 심전도 검사는 전에 받아 본 적이 있지만, 위내시경이나 소화기계 조영술은 전에 받아본 적이 없어요. 그러한 검사는 어떤 검사인가요?

효자: 위내시경과 상부 소화기계 조영술은 당신의 위를 검사하기 위한 것입니다. 위내시경은 의사가 당신의 입을 통해 긴 호수를 위까지 넣는 검사입니다.

미스 양: 아픈가요?

효자: 아니오, 호수를 삼킬 때 약간 불편한 감이 있지만 인후를 마취하기 위한 약을 투여할 것이기 때문에 전혀 아프지 않을 것입니다. 호수가 들어가면 의사가 당신의 식도, 위, 십이지장을 검사할 것입니다. 검사 받는 동안에는 긴장을 푸시는 것이 좋습니다. 원하신다면, 긴장완화를 돕기 위해 안정제를 드리겠습니다.

미스 양: 검사 때문에 긴장되니 안정제를 먹는 게 낫겠어요.
소화기계 조영술은 뭐죠?

효자: 음, 상부 소화기계 조영술은 당신의 위와 십이지장을 보기 위한 또 다른 검사방법입니다. 이 검사를 받을 때 바륨황산염을 마시게 되는데 이 바륨은 위를 코팅해서 엑스레이 상에서 위의 윤곽을 볼 수 있게 합니다. 그리고 나서 방사선 기사는 여러 장의 엑스레이 사진을 찍습니다. 하부 소화기계 조영술은 바륨 관장을 말합니다. 이 검사에서는 바륨을 관장을 통해 대장에 투여합니다. 엑스레이 상에 나타난 당신의 대장과 직장 윤곽을 보실 수 있습니다.

당신은 MRI검사를 받아야 합니다.

49 페이지

미스 양: 다른 검사도 받아야 합니까?

효자: 음, 혈압과 혈액 검사는 매일, 그리고 체온측정은 하루에 두 번씩 받으실 겁니다. 주치의가 검사 결과를 보고 나서 다른 검사 여부를 결정할 것입니다.

■ 다음 날

효자: 당신은 내일 아침 하부 소화기계 조영술을 받으실 겁니다. 오늘은 고형 음식을 드실 수 없습니다. 아침, 점심, 저녁에 묽은 수프와 쌀미음과 같은 유동식이 제공될 예정입니다. 제공 되는 것 외에는 아무것도 드시지 마세요.

미스 양: 쌀미음이 뭐죠?

효자: 쌀에 많은 양의 물을 넣어 아주 연해질 때까지 오랜 시간 동안 끓인 음식입니다.

미스 양: 아 그렇군요. 완화제를 먹어야 하나요?

효자: 예, 그렇습니다. 9시에 이 알약 두 개를 드시고 나서 아무 것도 마시거나 드시지 마세요.

UNIT 한글번역판

5 당신은 MRI검사를 받아야 합니다.

52 페이지

가로

1. 이 검사를 받기 위해서 환자는 검사 받을 컵에 소변의 일부를 받아야 합니다.
5. 이 검사에서는 사람의 정맥에서 혈액의 일부를 채취합니다.
7. 초음파 조영술, 메아리 혹은 초음파라고 불리우는 이 검사는 신체를 통과하는 소리의 음파를 통해 비정상적인 병변을 찾아내는 검사입니다.
10. 이 검사에서는 바륨 황산염이라 불리우는 물질이 관장을 통해 투여됩니다. 그리고 나서 대장과 직장의 많은 양의 엑스레이 사진을 찍습니다.
12. 이 검사는 의사가 환자의 시력을 검사합니다.

세로

2. 이 검사는 환자의 상완에 혈압측정띠를 둘러서 혈압을 측정하는 검사입니다.
3. EKG라고도 불리우는 이 검사는 의사가 전극을 환자의 흉부, 손목, 발목에 부착하여 심장상태를 알아보는 검사입니다.
4. 이 검사에서는, 계산된 단층 영상을 사용하여 신체 일부의 영상이 얻어 질 수 있습니다.
6. 검사에서는 의사가 인체에 길고 얇은 튜브를 삽입합니다. 의사는 신체의 내부를 들여다 볼 수 있고, 사진을 찍거나 조직의 일부를 채취할 수도 있습니다.
8. 뼈와 같은 신체의 내부의 사진을 찍기 위해 방사선을 이용하는 검사입니다.
9. 이 검사는 의사가 검사를 위해 신체 조직의 일부분 혹은 체액의 일부를 채취해서 현미경을 통해 비정상여부를 알아보는 검사입니다.
11. 이 검사에서 환자가 큰 통으로 된 기계에 들어가면 자기공명파가 신체를 뚫고 지나갑니다. 이러한 방법으로 신체내부의 사진을 얻습니다. 이 검사를 자기 공명 촬영술이라고도 합니다.

UNIT 5 당신은 MRI검사를 받아야 합니다.

53 페이지

역할 카드 A–간호사: 혈액 표본 채취

이해가 될 때까지 아래 지시사항을 여러 번 읽으시오; 그리고 나서 당신의 파트너와 역할극을 하십시오.

당신은 환자로부터 혈액표본을 채취하려고 합니다. 주사기와 진공채혈관을 준비하세요. 환자에게 의자에 앉은 후 팔걸이에 팔을 놓으라고 하세요. 주먹을 쥐라고 하세요. 지혈대로 환자의 팔 주위를 묶으세요. 알코올을 적신 솜으로 환자의 팔을 닦으세요. 주사바늘 뚜껑을 벗기세요. 환자에게 "약간 따끔합니다" 라고 말하세요. 주사 바늘을 환자의 정맥에 삽입하세요. 진공관을 밀어 넣어 혈액이 튜브안으로 들어가도록 하세요. 환자에게 주먹을 피라고 하세요. 환자의 팔에서 지혈대를 푸세요. 천자 부위에 알코올적신 솜을 대고 주사바늘을 제거하세요.

천자 부위에 반창고를 붙입니다. 환자에게 몇 분 동안 꾹 누르라고 하세요.

54 페이지

역할 카드 B–간호사: 호흡과 맥박 확인

이해가 될 때까지 아래 지시사항을 여러 번 읽으시오; 그리고 나서 당신의 파트너와 역할극을 하십시오.

당신은 환자로부터 호흡과 맥박을 확인하려고 합니다. 청진기를 준비하세요. 환자에게 호흡과 맥박을 확인하려고 한다고 말하세요. 환자에게 의자에 앉은 후 셔츠를 위로 올리라고 하세요. 청진기를 환자의 가슴에 올려 놓으세요. 환자에게 숨을 깊게 들이마시고 숨을 참으라고 하세요 환자에게 숨을 내쉬라고 하세요. 당신이 이곳 저곳을 청진하는 동안 몇 번 숨을 들이쉬고 내쉬라고 하세요. 환자에게 뒤로 돌라고 한 다음, 청진기를 환자의 등에 올려 놓으세요. 이곳 저곳을 청진하는 동안 몇 번 숨을 들이쉬고 내쉬라고 하세요. 검사가 끝나면 환자에게 셔츠를 내리라고 하세요. 다음은, 환자에게 맥박을 측정하려 한다고 말하세요. 당신의 손가락을 환자의 손목에 올려놓고 맥박을 측정하세요. 다 잰 후 환자에게 검사가 끝났다고 말하세요.

UNIT 6 당신은 임신했습니다.

55 페이지

연습1: 듣기 훈련

대화를 듣고 올바른 답을 고르세요.

1. 환자는 무엇을 하기 원합니까?
   a) 임신중절술을 받기 원한다.
   b) 임신반응검사를 받기 원한다.
   c) 피임약을 받기 원한다.
2. 사라는 그녀의 임신사실을 어떻게 알게 되었습니까?
   a) 그녀가 월경을 하지 않았다.
   b) 담당의사가 임신반응검사를 했다.
   c) 임시호르몬 반응검사에 양성결과가 나왔다.
3. 초경을 했을 때 환자의 나이는 몇 살이었습니까?
   a) 그녀는 17살이었다.
   b) 2년 전에
   c) 그녀는 12살이었다.
4. 환자는 어떤 검사를 받기 원합니까?
   a) 그녀는 임신반응검사를 받기 원한다.
   b) 그녀는 에치아이브이 검사를 받기 원한다.
   c) 그녀는 헤르프스 검사를 받기 원한다.

UNIT 6 당신은 임신했습니다.

58 페이지

연습3: 대화

대화를 듣고 밑줄에 들어갈 말을 채우세요.

■ 산부인과 병원에서

달: 축하합니다! 임신했다는 소식 들었습니다.

피셔: 감사합니다. 의사선생님께서 예정일이 9월 7일이라고 말씀하셨어요.

달: 이 책자는 산모와 아기를 위한 핸드북입니다. 한국에서는 "산모 수첩"이라고 합니다. 병원에 오실 때마다 가지고 오세요. 이 책자는 당신의 임신에 대한 기록이 될 것입니다. 또한, 아기가 태어난 후에는 아기의 건강상태와 예방접종에 대한 기록이 될 것입니다.

피셔: 정기 검진을 받으러 오면 주치의는 어떤 검사를 하시나요?

달: 주치의는 혈압, 소변검사, 체중체크를 합니다. 또한 아기의 발달상태를 확인하기 위해 내진과 초음파 검사도 합니다.

■ 34주 후,

달: 얼마마다 자국수축이 있습니까?

피셔: 5분 간격입니다.

달: 가운을 갈아입으세요. 이제 분만대기실로 갈 겁니다.

당신은 임신했습니다.

59 페이지

■ 분만실에서,

달: 자궁이 다 열렸습니다. 분만실로 갑시다.

닥터 선영: 아기의 머리가 보입니다. 힘주세요, 힘주세요. 좋아요, 자, 숨쉬세요. 다시 한 번 숨쉬세요. 자, 좋습니다. 힘주시고 좀 더 세게 힘주세요, 자 한번 더요. 됐습니다. 예쁜 따님을 얻으셨습니다.

달: 아기를 깨끗이 닦은 후 안겨 드리겠습니다. 여기에 있습니다.

■ 분만 후-피셔씨의 방

달: 아기가 울 때 마다 모유수유를 하실 수 있습니다. 모유수유 하기 전과 후에 몸무게를 재고 여기에 측정한 몸무게를 적어주세요. 수유가 끝나면 기저귀를 갈아주세요.

피셔: 아직 모유가 충분히 많지 않고, 색깔도 노란색이에요.

달: 처음에 나오는 모유를 “초유”라고 합니다. 초유는 아기한테 아주 좋습니다.

■ 퇴원 날

달: 아기는 대부분의 시간에 잠을 잡니다. 하지만 배고파서 밤에 자주 깰 수도 있습니다. 당신도 충분히 쉬도록 하세요.

피셔: 언제 검진을 받으러 다시 와야 합니까?

달: 4주 정도 후에 오세요. 하지만 아기한테 열, 설사, 호흡곤란, 경련, 황달과 같은 이상이 있으면 즉시 병원으로 오세요.

피셔: 알겠습니다. 도와주셔서 정말로 감사합니다.

당신은 임신했습니다.

62 페이지

연습4: 게임—당신의 유년 시절

당신이 어렸을 때

1. 위안을 주는 "안심 담요"가 있었습니까? 그것은 무엇이었습니까?
2. 아플 때 당신에게 안정감을 주는 "편안한 음식"으로 무엇이 있습니까?
3. 당신만의 특별한 장난감 혹은 책은 무엇이었습니까?
4. 유아원이나 유치원을 다녔습니까? 몇 살부터 다녔습니까?
5. 애완동물을 길렀습니까? 어떤 종류의 애완동물이었습니까?
6. 각별한 친구가 있었습니까?
7. 중병을 앓았습니까? 그것은 무슨 병이었습니까?
8. 입원했었습니까?

63 페이지

역할 카드 A—간호사

당신의 환자는 한국어를 못하는 외국인입니다. 서식을 채우기 위해 당신의 환자에게 질문하세요.

당신은 임신했습니다.

64 페이지

역할 카드 B—환자: 실비아 프랑코, 55세 여자

당신은 13세에 월경을 시작했습니다. 월경은 불규칙적이며, 마지막 월경은 3개월 전에 했습니다. 당신은 몇 달 간격으로 월경을 합니다.

당신은 세 아이가 있는데 24살, 26살 난 아들 둘과 16살 난 딸이 하나입니다. 첫 두 아이는 정상 분만을 했고, 딸은 제왕절개술로 분만을 했습니다.

당신은 피임 방법으로 콘돔을 사용합니다.

당신은 호르몬 대체 요법을 받기 위해 병원을 내원하기 원합니다. 당신의 문제는 성교시의 통증입니다. 이 증상은 약 3년간 있었습니다. 다른 증상은 작열감과 식은 땀입니다.

역할 카드 C—환자: 쥴리아 메이 북멘, 24세 여자

당신은 11세 6개월에 초경을 했습니다. 당신의 월경은 28일 간격으로 규칙적입니다. 당신의 마지막 월경은 2주 전에 했습니다. 당신은 한 번의 임신을 했었지만 5주 만에 유산되었습니다. 당신은 아이가 없습니다.

현재 당신은 피임 방법으로 콘돔을 쓰고 있지만 경구피임약으로 바꾸고 싶어 합니다. 당신은 경구피임약을 받기 위해 진료를 받기 원합니다. 당신은 다른 건강 문제나 증상은 없습니다.

UNIT 6

한글번역판

당신은 임신했습니다.

66 페이지

가로

3. 유산할 때 자궁경부를 확대하고 자궁을 긁어내는 시술
6. 태아를 밀어 내는 과정
7. 많은 임산부가 임신 초기에 경험하는 오심
8. 태어나기 전 엄마 뱃속의 아기
10. 임신의 인공 중절

12 여자들은 피임의 한 방법으로 이것을 먹는다.

13. 자궁과 질 사이에 있는 자궁의 아래 부위
14. 아기를 낳는 것
15. 의사가 자궁경부암 검사를 위해 여성 자궁경부의 일부 세포를 떼어내어 하는 검사
17. 콘돔과 같이 부부가 임신을 피하기 위해 하는 방법

세로

1. 자연 분만시 아기가 태어날 때 지나가는 생식 기관
2. 탯줄로 태아와 연결되어 있어 태아에게 음식을 전달해 주는 자궁 내막에 붙어 있는 장기
4. 출산시에 여자는 이것을 경험한다. 이것은 태아를 밀어 내도록 도와 준다.
5. 복부를 열어 아기를 출산하는 방법
7. 자발적인 임신의 중단
9. 아기를 분만하기 위한 특별 교육을 받은 간호사
11. 태아가 자라는 여성의 신체 부위
16. 신생아의 신체 상태를 체크하기 위한 검사 방법

우리 아기가 열이 납니다.

67 페이지

연습1: 듣기 훈련

대화를 듣고 올바른 답을 고르세요.

1. 메리는 얼마 동안 아팠습니까?
   a) 38.7도씨
   b) 3일 동안
   c) 하루 동안
2. 하워드는 언제 첫 디피티 예방접종주사를 맞았습니까?
   a) 3년 전에
   b) 일 년 전에
   c) 지난 주에
3. 라이언씨 딸은 어디가 아파서 왔습니까?
   a) 그녀는 구토증세가 있다.
   b) 그녀는 머리를 다쳤다.
   c) 그녀는 계속 울고 있다.
4. 아버지는 아들을 위해 무슨 예방 접종주사를 맞으러 왔습니까?
   a) 디프테리아, 백일해, 파상풍
   b) 일본 뇌염
   c) 홍역, 이하선염, 풍진

우리 아기가 열이 납니다.

70 페이지

연습3: 대화

대화를 듣고 밑줄에 들어갈 말을 채우세요.

■ 소아과에서

효진: 김도현?

아람: 예, 제 아들이 김도현입니다.

효진: 아드님은 몇 살입니까?

아람: 9개월 되었습니다.

효진: 어디가 아파 보입니까?

아람: 그는 신경질 적이고 힘이 없고 무기력해 보입니다. 또한 귀를 많이 만지곤 합니다.

효진: 열을 한번 재보겠습니다. 이 체온계를 아기의 겨드랑이 밑에 넣어 주세요. 이 전에 다른 질병이 있었습니까?

아람: 음, 그는 자주 감기에 걸리는 것 같습니다. 아기가 3개월 때쯤에 장미진에 걸렸었습니다.

효진: 도현에게 알러지가 있습니까? 특히나 약물에 대한 알러지가 있습니까?

아람: 약물에 대한 알러지는 없는 것 같지만 달걀에는 알러지가 있습니다.

효진: 좋습니다. 어디 보자. 열이 있네요. 체온이 38.5도입니다. 기다리시면 의사 선생님께서 곧 오실 겁니다.

우리 아기가 열이 납니다.

71 페이지

■ 잠시후에

아람: 의사선생님께서 도현의 귀에 염증이 있다고 하십니다. 항생제를 한 번 먹어 보고 염증이 낫지 않으면, 도현이를 이비인후과 전문의에게 보여주는 게 나을 것 같다고 하십니다.

효진: 여기 도현의 약이 있습니다. 이것은 항생제입니다. 가루약이므로 주스와 함께 섞어 먹일 수 있습니다. 이 약을 하루에 세 번 식사 후에 주세요. 이 노란 가루약은 해열제입니다. 이것은 아기 체온이 38도 이상 오를 때 주세요. 문의 사항이나 무슨 문제가 생기면 언제든지 전화주세요.

아람: 감사합니다. 사실, 도현의 예방 접종에 대해 몇 가지 여쭈어 볼 게 있습니다. 디피티, 소아마비, 결핵예방 주사는 5개월 때 맞았는데, 그 외에 맞아야 할 주사가 있습니까?

효진: 음, 디피티는 세 번, 소아마비는 두 번, 결핵 예방주사는 한 번 맞습니다.

아람: 알겠습니다. 그 외에 더 받아야 할 예방 접종이 있나요?

효진: 풍진, 홍역, 이하선염, 수두에 대한 예방 접종을 받아야 하는데, 아기가 만 1세가 되어야 접종할 수 있습니다. 아. 그리고 일본 뇌염 예방 접종도 있습니다.

아람: 그게 뭐죠?

효진: 모기에 의해서 감염되는 질환입니다. 자, 여기 영어로 되어 있는 예방 접종 계획표를 드리겠습니다.

아람: 감사합니다.

UNIT 7 한글번역판

우리 아기가 열이 납니다.

75 페이지

역할 카드 A–간호사

당신은 소아과에서 근무하는 간호사입니다. 수잔이라고 하는 소녀가 아버지와 함께 당신이 일하는 곳에 오고 있습니다.

하단의 서류를 작성하기 위한 질문을 소녀의 아버지께 하세요

소녀에게 피검사를 할 것이라고 말하세요. 그 후에 의사를 곧 만날 것이라고 소녀와 아버지에게 말하세요.

76 페이지

역할 카드 B–간호사

당신은 소아과에서 근무하는 간호사입니다. 빌리라고 하는 소년이 어머니와 함께 당신이 일하는 곳에 오고 있습니다.

하단에 있는 서류를 작성하기 위한 질문을 소년의 어머니께 하세요.

스미스씨는 소년에게 추가적으로 필요한 예방 접종에 대해 문의하고 있습니다. 소년이 받아야 할 예방 접종에 대해 설명하세요(힌트: 예방 접종표를 참고하세요).

홍역 접종을 받기 전에 빌리가 계란에 대해 알러지가 있다는 사실을 의사에게 알려야 한다고 빌리 어머니께 말하세요.

예방 접종 후에 빌리가 아프고 열이 나면 병원으로 데리고 오라고 빌리 어머니께 말하세요.

우리 아기가 열이 납니다.

77 페이지

역할 카드 C—환자의 아버지: 미스터 리

당신은 11살 난 딸, 수잔이 오른쪽 배에 콕콕 찌르는 심한 통증이 있어 병원으로 데리고 왔습니다. 복통은 이틀 정도 되었습니다. 그녀는 또한 오심과 열이 있습니다. 체온은 37. 8도 입니다.

수잔은 5살 때 기관지 폐렴을 앓았었습니다. 그녀는 약 3년 동안 천식을 앓고 있습니다. 그녀는 페니실린, 집 먼지, 진드기에 알러지가 있습니다.

77 페이지

역할 카드 D—환자의 어머니: 미즈 스미스

당신은 4살 난 아들, 빌리에게 수두 예방 접종을 하기 위해 병원으로 데리고 왔습니다. 그는 건강합니다. 체온은 36.5도 입니다.

빌리는 6개월 때 장미진을 앓았었습니다. 그는 종종 중이염을 앓곤 합니다. 만 1세에 처음으로 중이염에 걸렸습니다.

빌리는 계란에 알러지가 있습니다.

빌리는 다음과 같이 예방 접종을 받았습니다:

디피티—3회~2세에

비씨지—1회~9개월에

소아마비—2회~1세에

더 맞아야 할 예방 접종에 대해 간호사에게 물어보세요.

당신은 내일 오전 10시에 수술을 받을 예정입니다.

79 페이지

연습1: 듣기 훈련

대화를 듣고 올바른 답을 고르세요.

1. 에드워드씨는 수술 후 얼마 동안 병원에 입원해야 합니까?
   a) 일주
   b) 3주
   c) 2주
2. 스미스씨는 어떤 수술을 받아야 합니까?
   a) 췌장 수술
   b) 탈장 수술
   c) 담낭 수술
3. 호로비츠씨가 수술 받을 때는 어떤 종류의 마취시술을 받게 됩니까?
   a) 전신 마취
   b) 국소 마취
   c) 경막외 마취
4. 코토씨는 그녀가 필요한 물건들을 어디서 살 수 있습니까?
   a) 편의점에서
   b) 병원 매점에서
   c) 백화점에서

당신은 내일 오전 10시에 수술을 받을 예정입니다.

83 페이지

연습3: 대화

대화를 듣고 밑줄에 들어갈 말을 채우세요.

■ 수술 이틀 전 날

효자: 브라운씨, 당신의 위수술이 수요일 오전에 있을 예정입니다. 수술 전에 몇가지 준비하셔야 할 물품들이 있습니다.

브라운: 어떤 것들을 준비해야 합니까?

효자: 쇼핑백 2개, 목욕 타월 2개, 작은 타월 3개, 칫솔과 치약입니다. 또한 위수술을 받기 위해서는 좀 더 필요한 것들이 있습니다.

브라운: 더 필요한 것들이 뭐죠?

효자: 여기에 품목들이 있습니다. 병원 매점에서 이러한 물품들을 구입하실 수 있습니다.

브라운: 알겠습니다. 지금 가봐야겠군요.

효자: 이 물품들을 다 구입하시고 모든 물품에 지용성 잉크로 이름을 적은 후에 쇼핑백에 그 물품들을 담아 두세요.

■ 수술 하루 전

효자: 오늘은 바쁜 하루가 되겠어요. 오늘 오후에 마취과 전문의가 와서 당신이 시술 받을 마취에 대해 설명해 줄 겁니다. 그 후에 주치의가 수술에 대해 설명할 예정입니다.

브라운: 알겠습니다.

효자: 오늘 아침에는 간호사가 당신의 복부를 면도할 예정입니다. 면도가 끝나면, 몸을 씻으시고 머리를 감으세요.

브라운: 예.

효자: 오늘 저녁이 마지막 식사가 되겠습니다. 유동식이 제공 될 예정입니다. 자정까지 물이나 플레인 홍차는 마실 수 있습니다. 저녁 9시에 이 수면제를 드시길 바랍니다.

당신은 내일 오전 10시에 수술을 받을 예정입니다.

84 페이지

■ 수술 당일 날—수술 전

효자: 일어날 시간입니다, 브라운씨. 화장실 다녀오세요; 간호사가 관장할 예정입니다.

■ 조금 후에

효자: 브라운씨, 시계, 안경, 의치를 벗으세요. 모발 영양제는 쓰지 마세요. 욕실로 가셔서 이 수술 가운으로 갈아 입으시고 침상에서 쉬고 계세요.

브라운: 가운으로 갈아 입었습니다.

효자: 좋습니다. 당신의 방광에 도뇨관을 삽입할 겁니다. 그리고 나서 코를 통해 위장내관을 삽입할 예정입니다. 자, 이제 정맥 주사를 주입하겠습니다. 누군가 수술실로 당신을 모시러 올 때까지 쉬고 계세요.

■ 수술실에서

마취과 의사: 안녕하십니까, 브라운씨. 당신이 잠이 든 후에, 우리는 당신의 입을 통해 호흡기관을 삽일 할 겁니다. 자 이제 경막외 마취를 시행하겠습니다. 왼쪽으로 누우시고 최대한으로 허리를 구부리세요.

브라운: 이렇게요?

마취과 의사: 예, 좋습니다. 자, 다 됐습니다. 이제 똑바로 등을 대고 누우세요.

■ 수술 후—회복실에서

Dr. 양재준: 브라운씨, 수술이 끝났습니다. 모두 잘 되었습니다. 당신은 지금 회복실에 있습니다. 마취과 선생님께서 괜찮다고 하시면 곧 호흡기관을 빼고, 당신을 병동으로 보내드릴 겁니다.

당신은 내일 오전 10시에 수술을 받을 예정입니다.

87 페이지

역할 카드A－간호사

당신의 환자는 바바라 존스입니다. 그녀가 받을 수술에 대해 설명하세요.

수술의 종류: 유방 절제술

수술 날짜/시간: 목요일 아침

마취종류: 안정제, 전신마취

병원 입원 기간: 한 달

수술 전에 준비해야 할 물품: 목욕 타월 2개, 작은 타월 3개, 칫솔, 치약, 종이 쇼핑백 2개, 가운 1개, 면으로 된 티자바인더 1개, 속옷 한 벌, 주둥이가 달린 물컵 1개, 흉대 2개, 파자마 한 벌.

수술 전 날: 접착 테잎 검사, 복부, 흉부, 겨드랑이 면도, 목욕하기; 머리감기. 동의서에 서명하기. 수술 전 마지막 식사는 저녁에 일반식이 제공됨. 수면제 투약.

수술 날 아침: 아침 6시에 관장. 콘텍트 렌즈, 시계, 장신구 제거. 화장 불가. 수술 가운입고 수술 모자 쓰기. 도뇨관과, 위장내관 삽입 예정. 안정제 투약.

88 페이지

역할 카드 B－간호사

당신의 환자 이름은 제임스 스미스입니다. 그가 받아야 할 수술에 대해서 설명하세요.

수술 종류: 위 절제술

수술 날짜/시간: 화요일 오후

마취 종류: 경막외, 전신 마취

병원 입원 기간: 5주

수술 전에 준비해야 할 물품: 목욕 타월 2개, 작은 타월 3개, 칫솔, 치약, 종이 쇼핑백 2개, 가운 2벌, 복대 3개, 면으로 된 티자바인더 2개, 속옷 한 벌, 주둥이 달리 물컵 2개.

수술 전 날: 접착 테잎 검사, 흉부, 복부 면도. 목욕하기. 동의서에 서명. 마지막 식사가 유동식으로 저녁에 제공 됨.

수술날 아침: 오전 7시에 관장. 안경, 시계, 의치 제거. 모발 영양제는 사용불가. 수술실 가운으로 갈아입음. 도뇨관과 위장내관이 삽입될 예정. 정맥 주사 투입 예정.

당신은 내일 오전 10시에 수술을 받을 예정입니다.

89 페이지

역할 카드 C—환자

간호사의 지시를 듣고 그 혹은 그녀가 말하는 것을 점검해 보세요. 당신이 이해를 못 했거나 잘 못 들었으면 간호사에게 질문하세요.

수술 종류

[ ] 담낭 절제술 [ ] 위 절제술 [ ] 유방 절제술

[ ] 췌장 절제술 [ ] 소장 절제술

수술 날짜/시간

A: [ ] 월요일 [ ] 화요일 [ ] 수요일 [ ] 목요일 [ ] 금요일

B: [ ] 오전 [ ] 오후

마취 종류

[ ] 안정제 [ ] 국소 [ ] 경막외 [ ] 척추 [ ] 전신

입원 기간

A: [ ] 하루 [ ] 이틀 [ ] 사흘 [ ] 나흘 [ ] 닷새 [ ] 엿새

B: [ ] 일 [ ] 주 [ ] 달

수술 전 필요한 물품

[ ] 타월 [ ] 치약 [ ] 칫솔 [ ] 쇼핑백

[ ] 가운 [ ] 복대 [ ] 티자 바인더 [ ] 흉대

[ ] 속옷 [ ] 파자마 [ ] 주둥이가 달린 물컵

수술 전 날

[ ] 접착 테이프 테스트 [ ] 동의서에 서명 [ ] 목욕 하기`

[ ] 수면제 투약

면도 [ ] 겨드랑이 [ ] 복부 [ ] 흉부 [ ] 치골 부위 [ ] 목 근처

마지막 식사 A [ ] 아침식사 [ ] 점심식사 [ ] 저녁식사 B [ ] 일반식 [ ] 유동식

수술 당일 아침

[ ] 관장 [ ] 목욕 [ ] 수술 가운으로 갈아 입기

제거 [ ] 시계 [ ] 안경 [ ] 콘택트 렌즈 [ ] 장신구 [ ] 의치

사용 불가 [ ] 모발 영양제 [ ] 화장

삽입 예정인 물품 [ ] 좌약 [ ] 위장내관 [ ] 도뇨관 [ ] 정맥 주사

기분이 어떠십니까?

91 페이지

연습1: 듣기 훈련

대화를 듣고 올바른 답을 고르세요.

1. 존스씨의 문제는 무엇입니까?
   a) 그는 요통이 있다.　　b) 그는 배에 가스가 찼다.
   c) 그는 오심이 있다.　　d) 그는 열이 있다.
2. 애플비씨는 어제 식사량의 얼마를 먹었습니까?
   a) 그녀는 30%를 먹었다.　　b) 그녀는 50%를 먹었다.
   c) 그녀는 75%를 먹었다.　　d) 그녀는 100%를 먹었다.
3. 마리벨은 소변을 몇 회 보았습니까?
   a) 6회　　b) 넘버 원(배뇨)
   c) 3회　　d) 넘버 투(배변)
4. 실버스테인씨는 그녀의 약을 몇 번 먹어야 합니까?
   a) 130에 84
   b) 하루에 세 번 식전에
   c) 노란색 알약 2알과 핑크색 캡슐 한 알
   d) 하루에 세 번 식 후에

94 페이지

주의: 영어권 사람들은 소변과 대변 보는 것에 대해 직접적으로 말하지 않습니다. 미국에서는 화장실에 가야 할 경우에는 "휴게실/욕실/여성 전용 방/남성 전용 방/존(남성 전용 화장실)이 어디죠?" 라고 물을 것입니다. 영국에서는 "화장실/변소가 어디죠?" 라고 묻습니다.

어린 아이는 "배뇨하다" 와 "장의 움직임" 의 의미를 모를 수 있고, 용어를 아는 아이들은 그러한 용어를 쓸 때 당황해 할 수도 있습니다. 대부분 흔히, "넘버 원" 은 배뇨로 쓰이고, "넘버 투" 는 배변으로 쓰입니다. 어른들은 "나 쉬/똥 마려" 와 같은 좀 더 무례한 단어를 쓰기도 하지만, 친구 사이에서만 쓰고 병원에서는 전혀 쓰지 않습니다.

UNIT 9 기분이 어떠십니까?

95 페이지

연습3: 대화

대화를 듣고 밑줄에 들어갈 말을 채우세요.

■ 수술 후: 관찰실에서

로버트: 여기가 어디죠? 수술은 끝났나요?

효자: 수술이 끝났습니다. 당신은 지금 계시던 병동의 관찰실에 있습니다. 내일까지 여기에 있어야 합니다. 아프진 않으신가요?

로버트: 예, 오른쪽이 아픕니다.

효자: 진통제 주사를 하나 놔 드리겠습니다. 하지만 체온과 혈압을 먼저 확인해 보겠습니다. 좋습니다. 여기 진통제입니다. 잠을 자도록 해보세요.

■ 잠시 후

로버트: 목이 아주 마릅니다. 뭘 좀 마셔도 될까요?

효자; 메스꺼우신가요?

로버트: 예, 약간 그렇습니다.

효자: 음, 아직은 마실 수 없지만, 양치는 해도 됩니다. 양치질을 하면 좀 나아질 것입니다.

로버트: 알겠습니다.

■ 몇 시간 후에

효자: 기분이 어떠신가요?

로버트: 나아졌지만 통증이 약간 있습니다.

효자: 메스꺼우신가요?

로버트: 아니요. 전혀요.

UNIT 9

기분이 어떠십니까?

96 페이지

■ 다음 날 아침

효자: 안녕하세요, 로버트씨, 오늘 아침엔 어떠신가요?

로버트: 훨씬 좋아졌습니다.

효자: 회복이 아주 잘 되고 있습니다. 주치의가 도뇨관을 제거하면 병실로 가실 수 있습니다.

■ 로버트씨의 방

로버트: 오늘은 일어나도 되죠?

효자: 예, 운동을 빨리 시작할수록 치유속도가 빨라집니다. 하지만 처음에는 어지러울 수도 있으니 간호사에게 도움을 청하세요.

로버트: 화장실을 가야 합니다.

효자: 좋습니다. 천천히 일어나시고 발을 침대 옆쪽으로 내려 놓으세요. 천천히 일어나시고 제 팔을 잡으세요

■ 다음 날

효자: 여러분, 침대로 돌아가세요. 의사 선생님이 아침 회진을 돌고 있습니다.

닥터 민준: 간호사 선생님, 로버트씨의 상처부위를 열어주세요. 로버트씨, 치유가 잘 되고 있군요. 아마도 5일 정도 지나면 실밥을 제거할 수 있을 겁니다.

■ 이틀 후에

효자: 안녕하세요, 로버트씨. 여기에 약이 있습니다. 2캡슐을 하루에 세 번, 식사 후에 드세요.

UNIT 9

한글번역판

기분이 어떠십니까?

97 페이지

연습 4: 퍼즐–단어 순서가 뒤섞인 문장–일치 시키기

1. 정맥주사 투여가 끝났습니다.
2. 혈액을 채취하려고 합니다.
3. 항문에 좌약을 넣으려고 합니다.
4. 수술 가운으로 갈아입으세요.
5. 체온을 재세요.
6. 당신의 혈압은 150에 85입니다.
7. 관장을 하려고 합니다.
8. 요강이 필요한가요?
9. 주사를 놔야 합니다.
10. 상처부위 드레싱을 교환해야 합니다.
11. 의사 선생님이 내일 실밥을 뽑을 겁니다.
12. 엘리베이터를 타고 일층으로 가세요.
13. 이 컵에 소변의 일부를 받아 주세요.
14. 당신의 폐 소리를 듣겠습니다.
15. 메스꺼우신가요?
16. 화장실을 가야 한다면 간호사를 부르세요.

UNIT 9

기분이 어떠십니까?

100 페이지

역할 카드 A－간호사

당신의 환자는 제리 로페즈입니다. 그는 담낭 절제술을 받았습니다.

그에게 기분이 어떤지, 통증이 있는지, 식욕은 어떤지, 소변 대변은 보았는지 그리고 체온에 대해 질문하세요.

혈압을 잴 것이라고 그에게 말하세요. 혈압은 150에 95입니다. 로페즈씨에게 약을 주세요. 그는 하루에 한 번 자기 전에 흰색 알약 하나를 먹어야 합니다.

다음 페이지에 있는 일상 생활 기록지에 관련 정보를 기록하세요

역할 카드 B－간호

당신의 환자는 로젤리 갈리슨입니다. 그녀는 복부 탈장 제거술을 받았습니다.

그녀에게 기분이 어떤지, 통증이 있는지, 식욕은 어떤지, 소변 대변은 보았는지 그리고 체온에 대해 질문하세요.

혈액 채취를 할 것이라고 그녀에게 말하세요. 갈리슨씨에게 약을 주세요. 그녀는 하루에 세 번 식사 후에 파랗고 하얀 캡슐 하나를 먹어야 합니다.

다음 페이지에 있는 일상 생활 기록지에 관련 정보를 기록하세요.

101 페이지

역할 카드 C－환자

당신은 제리 로페즈입니다. 당신은 담낭 절제술을 받았습니다. 당신은 상태가 그리 좋지 않습니다; 당신은 메스꺼워서 지난 밤에 잠을 잘 수가 없었습니다. 당신은 허리에 통증이 있습니다. 식욕은 그리 좋지 않습니다. 당신은 어제 식사의 30% 정도만 먹었습니다. 당신은 대변은 보지 못했고, 소변은 7회 보았습니다. 당신의 체온은 37.9도입니다.

역할 카드 D－환자

당신은 로젤리 갈리슨입니다. 당신은 복부 탈장 제거술을 받았습니다. 당신은 기분이 그저 그렇습니다. 수술 부위가 매우 아픕니다. 식욕도 그저 그렇습니다. 당신은 식사의 60%를 먹었습니다. 당신은 대변을 한 번 보았고, 소변은 6회 보았습니다. 당신의 체온은 섭씨 36.8도 입니다.

걱정 되는 것이 있습니까?

103 페이지

연습1: 듣기 훈련

대화를 듣고 올바른 답을 고르세요.

1. 리베르만씨는 어떤 종류의 음식을 먹을 수 없습니까?
   a) 그녀는 치즈와 돼지고기를 먹을 수 없다.
   b) 그녀는 어떤 고기도 먹을 수 없다.
   c) 그녀는 갑각류와 돼지고기를 먹을 수 없다.
   d) 그녀는 어떤 식사도 할 수 없다.
2. 빌리는 왜 걱정하고 있습니까?
   a) 그는 꿰맨 부분이 가렵기 때문에 걱정하고 있다.
   b) 그는 그의 병이 잘 치유되지 않기 때문에 걱정한다.
   c) 그는 수술을 받을 예정이어서 걱정한다.
   d) 그는 의사가 실밥을 제거 할 때 아프지 않을까 걱정한다.
3. 제닝씨는 왜 수혈을 받기를 원하지 않습니까?
   a) 그녀는 에치아이브이에 감염될까봐 두려워 하기 때문에
   b) 그녀는 수술을 원하지 않기 때문에
   c) 그녀의 종교 때문에
   d) 그녀가 받을 수술에 대해 걱정하고 있기 때문에
4. 필립씨는 무엇을 원했습니까?
   a) 그는 진통제를 좀 더 원한다.
   b) 그는 집으로 돌아가기를 원한다.
   c) 그녀는 의사를 만나기를 원한다.
   d) 그녀는 모르핀을 끊기를 원한다.

걱정 되는 것이 있습니까?

106 페이지

연습3: 대화

대화를 듣고 밑줄에 들어갈 말을 채우세요.

■ 미국에서 온 간호사

효자: 안녕하세요, 저는 김효자입니다. 저희 병원에 오신 것을 환영합니다.

캐롤: 처음 뵙겠습니다. 제 이름은 캐롤 필립입니다.

효자: 한국에는 이번이 첫 방문이죠?

캐롤: 아니요, 대학교 시절에 한국에서 일 년 동안 교환학생으로 있었습니다.

■ 잠시 후

효자: 저희 병원에는 가끔 외국인 환자가 있습니다. 외국인 환자를 간호할 때 주의해야 할 점이 있나요?

캐롤: 미국에서는 다양한 민족, 종교, 문화적 배경을 가진 많은 환자들을 간호해야 합니다. 의사, 간호사들이 꼭 알아둬야 할 것은 그들간에는 서로 다른 차이가 있다는 것입니다.

효자: 가장 중요한 차이점이 뭐죠?

캐롤: 민족마다 의사, 병원, 치유에 대한 태도가 다르다는 점을 알아둬야 합니다. 예를 들면, 한국과 중국과 같은 어떤 민족들은 의사가 처방해 준 약과 함께 복용했을 때 어떤 부작용을 낫게 할 수 있는 한약을 복용합니다.

효자: 미국인 환자들에게 좀 특별히 챙겨야 할 것이 있나요?

캐롤: 제 생각에 미국인과 한국인과의 가장 큰 차이점은 미국인은 그들이 질병과 치료에 대한 모든 것에 대해 알고 싶어한다는 것입니다. 그들은 의사에게 질문을 많이 합니다.

효자: 예, 한국 환자들은 좀 더 수동적인 것 같네요.

캐롤: 또한 여러분이 고려해야 할 다른 한가지는 개인의 종교문제입니다. 예를 들면 카톨릭 신자가 있다면 그들은 죽기 전에 신부를 꼭 만나야 합니다.

걱정 되는 것이 있습니까?

107 페이지

어떤 종교는 수혈을 허락하지 않습니다. 또한 어떤 민족은 식이에 제한점이 있습니다. 이슬람이나 유대 민족들은 돼지 고기를 먹을 수 없습니다. 그래서 개인의 종교를 알아내고, 그들에게 어떤 제한 사항이나 특별한 요구 사항이 있는지를 물어봐야 합니다.

효자: 종교를 알아둬야 하는 것이 그렇게 중요한 것인지 몰랐었습니다. 음, 당신과 얘기를 나눌수 있어서 좋았습니다. 말이 난 김에 말씀 드리는데, 제가 일하는 병동에 영국인이 한 명 있습니다. 당신이 그와 함께 대화를 나누면 아주 좋을 것 같습니다.

■ 병동에서

효자: 윌슨씨, 이 분은 캐롤 필립스입니다. 그녀는 미국에서 방문한 간호사입니다.

윌슨: 처음 뵙겠습니다. 만나서 반갑습니다.

캐롤: 잘 지내시나요? 한국에서의 병원생활에 어떤 어려운 점이 있나요?

윌슨: 음, 효자씨와 제 주치의가 영어를 잘 해서 저는 정말 좋습니다.

캐롤: 걱정이나 염려되는 점은 없습니까?

윌슨: 솔직히 말씀 드리면, 제가 받게 될 수술에 대해 걱정이 됩니다. 제가 그 수술을 꼭 받아야 하는지에 대해 궁금합니다. 서양에서 우리는 항상 2차소견을 받아 보지만, 한국에서는 그러한 것은 관습에 어긋납니다.

108 페이지

캐롤: 예, 당신의 걱정이 이해가 가는군요. 아마도, 당신의 주치의와 다시 한번 상의하셔야 할것 같습니다. 주치의를 만날 때 제가 같이 해도 되겠습니까? 아마도 당신이 이해하지 못하는 것에 대해 설명을 해드릴 수 있을 겁니다.

윌슨: 예, 당신이 함께 하면 좋겠군요. 주치의가 오늘 저녁 8시에 들를 거라고 했어요.

캐롤: 8시 전에 꼭 다시 오겠습니다.

윌슨: 필립양, 대화를 나눌 수 있어서 기뻤습니다.

■ 간호사 라운지에서

효자: 당신이 윌슨씨와 말씀을 나눴다니 기쁩니다. 저는 그분이 얼마나 걱정하고 있는지 깨닫지 못했습니다.

캐롤: 도와드릴 수 있어서 기뻤습니다.

효자: 이제는 저도 환자분께 그분의 염려나 바라는 바를 직접 물어보는게 최선의 방법이라는걸 깨달았습니다.

걱정 되는 것이 있습니까?

109 페이지

연습4: 퍼즐

1. 어느 것이 가장 오래된 종교입니까?
   a) 부다교　b) 유대교　c) 힌두교
2. 어느 종교가 가장 많은 신도를 갖고 있습니까?
   a) 부다교　b) 크리스트교　c) 무슬림
3. 어느 사람들이 약초(한약)를 사용합니까?
   a) 중국인　b) 아메리카 원주민　c) 한국인
4. 어느 종교가 쇠고기 먹는 것을 금지하고 있습니까?
   a) 유다교　b) 무슬림　c) 힌두교
5. 어느 나라가 사람의 머리를 만지는 것이 그 사람의 영혼을 데려가 버릴 수 있다고 믿습니까?
   a) 베트남　b) 일본　c) 폴란드
6. 어느 종교가 담배 피우는 것과 수혈을 금지하고 있습니까?
   a) 신도(神道)　b) 여호와의 증인　c) 유대교
7. 어느 종교가 낙태와 이혼을 금지하고 있습니까?
   a) 유대교　b) 캐톨릭　c) 불교
8. 어느 종교가 자살을 금지하고 있습니까?
   a) 불교　b) 이슬람　c) 캐톨릭
9. 어느 종교에서 남자아기들이 태어난 직후 할례를 받습니까?
   a) 크리스트교　b) 불교　c) 유대교
10. 어느 종교에서 여성들은 아기를 낳기 위해서는 의사나 조산원이 여자여야 합니까?
    a) 불교　b) 유대교　c) 무슬림

걱정 되는 것이 있습니까?

110 페이지

역할 카드 A–간호사

서식을 채우기 위해 당신의 환자에게 질문하세요.

당신의 환자는 무슬림이고 돼지고기를 먹을 수 없습니다.

그는 그의 질병치료에 필요한 인슐린이 돼지의 췌장에서 만들어 진다는 것에 대해 걱정하고 있습니다.

당신이 그의 문제를 그의 의사에게 설명하고 그들이 돼지 대신에 양이나 소로부터 얻은 인슐린을 사용할 수 있는지 알아보겠다고 그에게 말하세요.

역할카드 B–간호사

서식을 채우기 위해 당신의 환자에게 질문하세요.

당신의 환자는 매우 늙고 혼자서 걸을 수 없습니다.

그녀의 침대 옆에 간이 변기를 갖다 놓을 것이고 간호사가 그녀의 변기 사용을 도울 것이라고 당신의 환자에게 말하세요.

당신의 환자는 정말로 수술이 필요한지 걱정하고 있습니다. 당신이 그녀의 의사에게 그녀의 궤양 치료를 위해 수술이외의 방법이 있는지 물어보겠다고 그녀에게 말하세요.

걱정 되는 것이 있습니까?

112 페이지

역할카드 C – 환자: 압둘 모하메드, 46세 남성

당신은 당뇨병이 있어 입원하였습니다.

당신은 이집트인이고 당신의 종교는 무슬림입니다. 당신의 종교는 돼지를 먹는 것을 허락하지 않습니다.

당신은 4인실에서 지내고 싶어합니다.

당신은 고혈압약을 복용중입니다.

당신은, 당신이 당뇨의 치료를 위해 인슐린을 써야만 하고 인슐린이 돼지의 췌장에서 만들어 진다는 것을 들었기 때문에 걱정하고 있습니다.

당신은 돼지의 어느 부분이라도 당신의 몸 안에 받아들일 수 없습니다.

역할카드 D – 환자: 순 웨이 린, 85세 할머니

당신은 위궤양으로 수술을 받기 위해 입원하였습니다.

당신은 중국인이고 종교는 불교입니다. 당신은 당신의 종교로 인한 특별한 제한은 없습니다.

당신은 혼자 걸을 수 없고, 그래서 휠체어를 사용합니다.

당신은 일인실에서 지내고 싶어합니다.

당신은 많은 종류의 한약을 복용중입니다.

당신은 수술하는 것을 정말 겁내고 있습니다. 당신은 나이가 아주 많기에, 당신이 정말로 그걸 꼭 해야 하는지에 대해 궁금해하고 있습니다.

Transcripts and Answers

UNIT 1 Do you work on the surgical ward?

Activity 1: Listening Practice (CD 2)

1. Tomas: Could you tell me your name please?
   Delores: My name is Delores Agosto.
   Tomas: Could you spell your family name?
   Delores: D－E－L－O－R－E－S
   Tomas: And could you spell you family name?
   Delores: A－G－O－S－T－O
   Tomas: Could you speak more slowly?
   Delores: sure, A－G－O－S－T－O
   A: C) Agosto
2. Jihye: Where do you live?
   Mr. green: I live in Seoul. Do you want my address?
   Jihye: No, but I would like your phone number.
   Mr. green: It's 02－6299－8614.
   Jihye: Could you say that again please?
   Mr. green: 02－6299－8614.
   Jihye: Did you say 8641 or 8614?
   Mr. green: I said 8614.
   A: a) 02－6299－8614.
3. Dal: What do you do?
   Enrique: I'm talking with you.
   Dal: No, I mean, What's your occupation?
   Enrique; I'm sorry, What is the meaning of occupation?
   Dal: It means job. What is your job?
   Enrique: Oh, I'm an X－ray technician.
   A: b) She wants to know his occupation.
4. Elie: Dr. Minjun, this is Harvey Jones. She's a nurse in the psychiatric department. Harvey, this is Dr. Minjun Kim. He's an obstetrician.
   Harvey: How do you do?
   Dr. Minjun: It's really nice to meet you.
   Harvey: I'm sorry, I didn't get your name, doctor.
   Dr. Minjun: It's Kim Minjun. My family name is spelled K－I－M.
   Harvey: I see. Thank you.
   A: b) He's a nurse.

Activity 3: Dialog (CD 4)

1. introduce
2. How do you do
3. Please don't hesitate
4. rounds
5. nurses' lounge
6. This is
7. ward
8. show you the ropes
9. are you from
10. nursing school
11. you are my senior
12. near this hospital
13. hobbies
14. great idea

Activity 4: Puzzle

1. obstetrics
2. internal medicine
3. dentistry
4. pediatrics
5. radiology
6. gynecology
7. cardiology
8. plastic surgery
9. opthalmology
10. rehabilitation
11. psychiatry
12. dermatology
13. anesthesiology
14. orthopedics
15. neurology
16. oral surgery

UNIT 2 What's seems to be the problem today?

Activity 1: Listening Practice (CD 5)

1. Hyoja: Is this your first visit?
Mr. Wong: Yes, it is.
Hyoja: Do you have an insurance card?
Mr. Wong: No, I don't
Hyoja; What department do you want to visit?
Mr. Wong: Well, I'm suffering from lower back pain, so I think I should go to the orthopedics department.
A: b) He's got lower back pain.

2. Hyoja: What's your problem today, Mrs. Jefferson?
Mrs. Jefferson: I've been feeling sick for two days.
Hyoja: What are your symptoms?
Mrs. Jefferson: I have a cough and diarrhea.
Hyoja: Do you have a fever?
Mrs. Jefferson: Yes, my temperature is 38°.
A: b) She has a fever, diarrhea and a cough.

3. Hyoja: What department would you like to visit?
Ms. Goldberg: Well, I'm not sure.
Hyoja: What seems to be the problem?
Ms. Goldberg: I found a lump in my breast.
Hyoja: Then, I think you had better go to the surgical department.
A: b) Surgery

4. Hyoja: Mr. Jones, how have you been feeling?
Mr. Jones: I haven't been feeling well recently.
Hyoja: What's the matter?
Mr. Jones: I've had stomach pain and heartburn.
Hyoja: How long have you had these symptoms?
Mr. Jones: I've been having pain for about two months and I often get heartburn in the evening.
Hyoja: Have you had any nausea or vomiting?
Mr. Jones: Yes, this past week I've been nauseous every day.
A: c) For two months.

Activity 3: Dialog (CD 7)

1. Have you visited
2. fill in this form
3. Could you spell
4. height
5. weigh
6. I'm 55years old
7. your problem
8. suffering from
9. How long
10. about 3 or 4
11. Almost every day
12. with your heart
13. when I was a patient
14. will see you

Activity 4: Puzzle

9, 8, 3, 11, 4, 7, 2, 6, 1, 10, 5

UNIT 3 This is the nurses' station.

Activity 1: Listening Practice (CD 8)

1. Hyoja: Visiting hours are from 1 to 7 on weekdays and from 11 to 7 on Saturdays and Sundays.
   Mr. Martin: I see. What time is lunch served?
   Hyoja: At noon.
   A: c) from 11 to 7
2. Hyoja: This is the bath. Men can use it on Monday, Wednesday and Friday and women can use it on Tuesday, Thursday and Saturday.
   Mr. Martin: Can I take a bath this morning?
   Hyoja: No, the hours are from 2 to 5 in the afternoon. You will need to take a bath before your surgery or before some tests. A nurse will tell you when you can use it.
   A: c) Tuesday, Thursday, Saturday
3. Mr. Martin: Can I eat my meals in my own room?
   Hyoja: Patients who can walk should go to the dining room for their meals. After surgery or if you need rest, your meals will be brought to your room.
   Mr. Martin: What time are the meals?
   Hyoja: Breakfast is at 7:30am, lunch at noon and dinner at 6pm.
   A: c) dining room
4. Hyoja: This is the nurse call button by your bed. If you need a nurse's assistance, please push this button. There is also a nurse call button in the bath and in the toilet.
   Mr. Martin: Where is the toilet?
   Hyoja: It's down the hall on the left.
   A: c) toilet, bath, patient's bed

Activity 3: Dialog (CD 10)

1. nurse
2. head nurse
3. clothes
4. bedside table
5. change into your pajamas
6. around the ward
7. nurses' station
8. Across from
9. in the lobby
10. The toilets are
11. wash your face
12. What's in this room
13. from 9am to 6pm
14. on your left

Activity 4: Puzzle 1

A: examination room
B: laundry
C: dining room
D: consultation room
E: bath

Activity 4: Puzzle 2

(8) baby bottle
(5) bedpan
(14) blood pressure gauge
(3) cast
(21) crutches
(11) diaper
(17) emesis(kidney) basin
(2) examination table
(19) gauze
(6) IV drip
(20) latex gloves
(12) medical chart
(23) microscope
(24) nurse call button
(7) oxygen
(15) scale
(1) sling
(25) spouted water cup
(18) stethoscope
(9) stretcher
(22) syringe(needle)
(13) thermometer
(16) vital signs monitor
(10) walker
(4) X-ray

UNIT 4 Are you suffering from any illnesses?

Activity 1: Listening Practice (CD 11)

1. Hyoja: Ms. Cane, could you tell me your next of kin or someone we can contact in case of emergency?
   Ms. Cane: Minjun Kim.
   Hyoja: Whats's his relationship to you?
   Ms. Cane: He's my husband.
   Hyoja: Could you tell me his phone number at work and at home?
   Ms. Cane: Our home number is 741−4494 and his work number is 762−9194.
   A: c) He is Ms. Cane's husband.
2. Hyoja: What is your regular diet, Ms. Cane?
   Ms. Cane: Well, I eat 3 meals a day, plus a snack in the afternoon. I try to eat a balanced diet.
   Hyoja: Do you have any restrictions in your diet?
   Ms. Cane: Yes, I eat a low−salt diet because of my hypertension.
   Hyoja: I see. Do you eat rice at every meal?
   Ms. Cane: I eat rice once or twice a day.
   A: b) She doesn't eat very salty food.
3. Hyoja: Do you smoke?
   Ms. Cane: Now, I don't. But I used to smoke. I smoked for 7 years, but I quit 2 years ago.
   Hyoja: Do you drink alcohol?
   Ms. Cane: A little. I drink a glass of wine or beer every day.
   A: b) She drinks a glass every day.
4. Hyoja: Could you tell me your family history? Are your parents alive?
   Ms. Cane: My mother is alive. She suffers from diabetes. My father passed away 5 years ago. He had a heart attack. I have a younger brother and older sister. My sister also has hypertension. My brother is healthy.
   Hyoja: Do you have any children?
   Ms. Cane: Yes, I have 2 daughters, age 19 and 23 and a son, age 17.
   A: a) He had a heart attack.

Activity 3: Dialog (CD 13)

1. hospital
2. admission
3. my right side
4. hypertension
5. suffering from
6. Have you ever
7. I'm taking
8. your doctor
9. allergies
10. daily activities
11. bathtub
12. vision and hearing
13. personality
14. worried about
15. can speak English

Activity 4: Puzzle

U	A	A	C	A	T	A	R	A	C	T	Q	R	E	A
W	X	S	P	L	E	U	K	E	M	I	A	S	M	F
H	L	E	T	P	K	S	S	N	A	A	A	E	F	X
S	A	P	T	H	E	A	E	D	B	E	Z	D	R	E
I	S	I	B	U	M	N	H	Y	S	C	B	U	A	E
S	I	L	R	B	O	A	D	I	E	Y	X	P	C	N
O	T	E	E	V	B	G	D	I	Q	X	V	A	T	O
L	I	P	D	A	L	T	A	V	C	R	M	J	U	T
U	L	S	E	H	R	I	J	M	D	I	B	M	R	S
C	L	Y	V	A	D	P	O	L	P	S	T	L	E	L
R	I	G	E	S	C	B	M	T	L	Z	E	I	Y	L
E	S	H	D	I	A	B	E	T	E	S	P	V	S	A
B	N	H	E	P	A	T	I	T	I	S	L	U	I	G
U	O	K	M	M	S	I	L	O	H	O	C	L	A	H
T	T	L	N	O	I	S	N	E	T	R	E	P	Y	H

1. 천식
2. 후천성면역결핍증
3. 알콜중독
4. 맹장염
5. 백내장
6. 당뇨
7. 습진
8. 간질
9. 골절
10. 담석
11. 통풍
12. 심질환
13. 간염
14. 두드러기
15. 고혈압
16. 백혈병
17. 편도선염
18. 결핵

UNIT 5 You need to have an MRI.

Activity 1: Listening Practice (CD 14)

1. Hyoja: I need to take a blood sample, Ms. Smith.
   Ms. Smith: All right.
   Hyoja: Could you please put your arm here and make a fist? OK, you can relax now. Have you ever had any problems with your blood clotting?
   Ms. Smith: No, I haven't.
   Hyoja: OK, please apply pressure for 3 minutes.
   A: b) taking a blood sample.
2. Hyoja: Mr. Silver, before your surgery, you need to have a blood test, urine test, lung function test and an ECG.
   Mr. Silver: Should I have the tests today or after I'm admitted?
   Hyoja: You should have the tests after your admission.
   A: d) after his admission
3. Hyoja: Ms. Jackson, your doctor said you need to have a gastroscopy.
   Ms. Jackson: I never had one before. What is it?
   Hyoja: The doctor inserts a long tube with a lens into your stomach through your mouth. He can examine your stomach with it.
   Ms. Jackson: I see.
   A: b) her stomach
4. Hyoja: Mr. Kim, you need to have an MRI. Please take this elevator to the first floor. Turn right and go to the X−ray department: that's window 30.
   Mr. Kim: I should go to the first floor, then turn right and go to window 30.
   Hyoja: Yes, that's right. Just give them this form.
   A: a) an RI

Activity 3: Dialogs (CD16)

1. some tests
2. X−ray
3. chest
4. your stomach
5. a little
6. be painful
7. about the tests
8. lining
9. need to have
10. take your temperature
11. tomorrow morning
12. Please take

Activity 4: Crossword Puzzle

ACROSS
1. URINALYSIS
5. BLOOD TEST
7. ECHOGRAM
10. BARIUM ENEMA
12. EYE TEST

DOWN
2. BLOOD PRESSURE TEST
3. ELECTROCARDIOGRAM
4. CT SCAN
6. ENDOSCOPY
8. X−RAY
9. BIOPSY
11. MRI

UNIT 6 You're going to have a baby!

Activity 1: Listening Practice (CD 17)

1. Dal: What's the purpose of your visit?
   Mary: I think I'm pregnant.
   Dal: When was your last period?
   Mary: About 6 weeks ago.
   Dal: OK, we'll give you a pregnancy test.
   A: b) She wants a pregnancy test.
2. Dal: What's your problem today, Sarah?
   Sarah: I'm pregnant and I want to have an abortion.
   Dal: Did you have a pregnancy test?
   Sarah: Yes, I did a home pregnancy test and it was positive.
   A: c) Her home pregnancy test was positive.
3. Dal: When did you start menstruating?
   susan: When I was 12years old.
   Dal: when was your last period?
   susan: It began 2 weeks ago, on May 17th.
   A: c) She was 12 years old.
4. Ms. Grimes: I'd like to be tested for HIV.
   Dal: All right, just take a number and wait for a few minutes.
   Ms. Grimes: When can I get the results of the test?
   Dal: Come back in one week. Don't forget to bring your number
   A: b) She wants an HIV test.

Activity 3: Dialog (CD 19)

1. to have a baby
2. Please bring it with you
3. kinds of tests
4. Every 5 minutes
5. labor
6. let's go to
7. push harder
8. before and after
9. it's color is
10. good for the baby
11. sleep most
12. if your baby has any problems

Activity 6: Crossword Puzzle

ACROSS
3. D&C
6. LABOR
7. MORNING SICKNESS
8. FETUS
10. ABORTION
12. PILL
13. CERVIX
14. DELIVERY
15. PAP SMEAR
17. BIRTH CONTROL

DOWN
1. VAGINA
2. PLACENTA
4. CONTRACTIONS
5. CESAREAN SECTION
6. MISCARRIAGE
9. MIDWIFE
11. UTERUS
16. APGAR SCORE

UNIT 7 My baby has a fever.

Activity 1: Listening Practice (CD 20)

1. Hyojin: What's Mary's problem today?
   Mrs. Arthur: I think she has a stomach virus.
   Hyojin: What are her symptoms?
   Mrs. Arthur: She's been vomiting and has diarrhea.
   Hyojin; How long has she had these symptoms?
   Mrs. Arthur: Since around noon yesterday.
   Hyojin; Does she have a fever?
   Mrs. Arthur: Yes, her temperature was 38.7° this morning.
   Hyojin: Let's check her temperature now, please put this thermometer under her armpit.
   A: b) for 1 day
2. Hyojin: Hello, Mrs. Fisher. How is Howard feeling today?
   Mrs. Fisher: He's fine. We're here for this DPT booster.
   Hyojin: When did he have his first shot?
   Mrs. Fisher: It's right here in the Maternal and Child Health Handbook. A little over a year ago.
   Hyojin: Does he have a fever or has he been feeling sick this past week?
   Mrs. Fisher: No, he's been very healthy recently.
   A: b) over a year ago
3. Hyojin: Ms. Ryan, what's the matter with your daughter?
   Ms. Ryan: She fell and hit her head.
   Hyojin: How far did she fall?
   Ms. Ryan: About a meter.
   Hyojin: Has she had any unusual symptoms, like vomiting?
   Ms. Ryan: No, she didn't vomit.
   Hyojin: OK, Just wait here and we'll X−ray her head right away.
   A: b) She hit her head.
4. Hyojin: What is the purpose of your visit today?
   Mr. Jones: I'd like my son, Alan, to have a vaccination.
   Hyojin: What kind of vaccination does he need?
   Mr. Jones: I'd like him to have an MMR vaccination.
   Hyojin: We don't give measles, mumps and rubella in one injection in Korea. He'll have to have each one separately.
   Mr. Jones: I see. So what should I do?
   Hyojin: Why don't we give him the measles vaccine today and you can come back for the other two vaccinations.
   Mr. Jones: OK. That's what I'll do.
   A: c) Measles, mumps and rubella

Activity 3: Dialog (CD 22)

1. My son is
2. to be the problem
3. his ear
4. under his armpit
5. have any allergies
6. does have a fever
7. is suffering from
8. you can mix it
9. If you have any questions
10. What else
11. other inoculations
12. What's that

Activity 4: Puzzle

E	M	M	I	P	S	E	L	S	A	E	M
D	N	U	M	O	R	N	U	D	X	O	O
I	P	C	M	R	W	N	E	L	G	I	C
P	S	T	E	P	S	O	D	B	L	H	X
H	I	E	U	P	S	T	I	O	I	H	L
T	S	T	M	Z	H	F	P	C	X	X	F
H	S	A	J	D	O	A	K	O	A	X	X
E	U	N	G	Y	D	E	L	A	X	A	H
R	T	U	P	P	N	C	G	I	G	T	Q
I	R	S	T	P	N	L	J	I	T	C	U
A	E	G	O	F	A	D	W	J	D	I	B
J	P	X	V	A	L	L	E	B	U	R	S

3. 백일해
4. 풍진
5. 수두
6. 유행성 이하선염
7. 소아마비
8. 파상풍
9. 디프테리아
10. 홍역

UNIT 8 Your surgery will be tomorrow at 10am.

Activity 1: Listening Practice (CD 23)

1. Mr. Edwards: What kind of surgery do I need?
   Hyoja: You need to have a hernia removed from your abdomen, Mr. Edwards.
   Mr. Edwards: How long will I have to stay in the hospital?
   Hyoja; About two weeks. first, you need to have tests, then you need about a week for your recovery from the surgery.
   A: a) one week

2. Hyoja: Ms. Smith, how are you doing today?
   Ms. Smith: I'm nervous about my gallbladder operation.
   Hyoja: Gallbladder sugery is one of the easiest operations. These days the surgeon does it using a camera making just 3 small slits. The recovery time is very quick and there is little post－op pain.
   Ms. Smith: I'm relieved to hear that.
   A: c) gallbladder surgery

3. Mr. Horowitz: I'm having anal surgery tomorrow, and I'm wondering what kind of anesthesia they'll use.
   Hyoja: The anesthesiologist will come and talk to you later about your anesthesia, Mr. Brown.
   Mr. Horowitz: Do you thik they'll use general anesthesia? I don't want to be awake during my operation.
   Hyoja: These days they use many kinds of anesthesia, general, epidural, spinal, local. But don't worry! They'll use general anesthesia so you'll be asleep when they perform your operation.
   A: a) general anesthesia

4. Hyoja: Ms. Young, you need to prepare some things before your surgery.
   Ms. Cotto: What kinds of thing?
   Hyoja: You need some towels, a toothbrush and toothpaste and 2 paper shopping bags.
   Ms. Cotto: That's a lot of things; let me write it down. OK, anything else?
   Hyoja: Yes, for breast surgery, you also need a gown which opens in the front, 1 cotton T－binder, a pair of underpants, 2 chest binders, a pair of pajamas and a spouted water cup.
   Ms. Cotto: Where can I get these things?
   Hyoja: At the hospital shop. Just show them this list.
   Ms. Cotto: Oh, that's very convenient.
   A: b) at the hospital shop

Activity 3: Dialog (CD 26)

1. Wednesday morning
2. shopping bags
3. write your name
4. your doctor will talk with you
5. take a bath
6. You can drink water
7. Please go to the toilet
8. remove your watch
9. operating room
10. lie on your left side
11. your surgery is over

Activity 4: Puzzle

(27) appendix 맹장
(20) bladder 방광
(9) bone 뼈
(8) brain 뇌
(19) duedenum 십이지장
(11) esophagus 식도
(16) gallbladder 담낭
(29) heart 심장
(24) kidney 신장
(28) large intestine 대장
(6) liver 간
(1) lung 폐
(10) ovary 난소
(21) pancreas 췌장
(3) penis 음경
(13) prostate 전립선
(22) rectum 직장
(25) rib 갈비뼈
(2) small intestine 소장
(17) spleen 비장
(7) stomach 위
(23) testicle 고환
(26) throat 목구멍
(15) thyroid 갑상선
(4) tonsil 편도
(18) ureter 요관
(5) uterus 자궁
(14) uvula 목젖
(12) vagina 질

UNIT 9 How are you feeling?

Activity 1: Listening Practice

1. Hyoja : Mr. Jones, how are you feeling?
   Mr. Jones: I'm not feeling so good.
   Hyoja: What's the matter?
   Mr. Jones: I couldn't sleep very well last night.
   Hyoja: Are you feeling any pain?
   Mr. Jones: Yes, my abdominal area is very painful.
   Hyoja: It's probably gas. Let me listen to your intestines. Yes, you have a lot of intestinal movement. Getting out of bed and walking will help you get rid of the gas.
   A: b) He has gas.
2. Hyoja: Good morning. Ms. Appleby. How are you feeling?
   Ms. Appleby: I'm feeling pretty good.
   Hyoja: What's your temperature?
   Ms. Appleby: It's 37°.
   Hyoja; How was your appetite yesterday?
   Ms. Appleby: It was good. I ate about 3/4 of my meals.
   A: c) She ate 75%.
3. Hyoja: Good morning. Maribel. How are you feeling today?
   Maribel: Good morning. Ms. Kim. I'm feeling fine.
   Hyoja: Maribel, yesterday, how many times did you move your bowels?
   Maribel: I don't understand "bowels".
   Hyoja: It means number 2. How many times did you do number 2?
   Maribel: Let me see, 3 times.
   Hyoja: OK, and how many times did you urinate?
   Maribel: Does that mean number 1?
   Hyoja: Yes.
   Maribel: I did number 1, I think 6 times.
   A: a) 6 times.
4. Hyoja: How are you feeling today, Ms. Silverstein?
   Ms. Silverstein: I'm feeling much better.
   Hyoja: I'm glad to hear that. I need to take your blood pressure.
   Ms. Silverstein: How is my blood pressure?
   Hyoja: It's good. It's 130 over 84. Here's your medication. This is for one day.
   Ms. Silverstein: When should I take it?
   Hyoja: Please take 2 yellow tablets and I pink capsule, 3 times a day after meals.
   Ms. Silverstein: I take 2 yellow tablets and I pink capsule, 3 times a day after meals.
   Hyoja: Yes, that's right.
   A: d) 3times a day after meals.

Activity 3: Dialog (CD 29)

1. Where am I
2. your temperature
3. I have something
4. brush your teeth
5. I have some pain
6. feeling much better
7. The doctor will
8. may feel dizzy
9. sit up slowly
10. to your beds
11. in five days
12. your medicine

Activity 4: Puzzle

Scrambled Sentences

1. Your drip is finished.
2. I'm going to take a blood sample.
3. I'm going to insert a suppository into your anus.
4. Please change into this surgical gown.
5. Please take your temperature.
6. Your blood pressure is 150 over 85.
7. I'm going to give you an enema.
8. Do you need use the bedpan?
9. I need to give you an injection.
10. I have to change your dressing on the wound.
11. The doctor will remove your stitches tomorrow.
12. Take the elevator to the first floor.
12. Please put a urine sample in this cup.
14. I want to listen to your lungs.
15. Do you feel nauseous?
16. Please call a nurse if you need to go to the toilet. (If you need to go to the toilet, please call a nurse)

Matching

A) 8	G) 10	M) 14
B) 3	H) 4	N) 9
C) 11	I) 12	O) 7
D) 16	J) 1	P) 2
E) 5	K) 13	
F) 15	L) 6	

UNIT 10 Are you worried about anything?

Activity 1: Listening Practice (CD 30)

1. Jihye: Hello, Mrs. Lieberman, I'm Jihye kim. I'm going to be your nurse.
   Mrs. Lieberman: Oh, hello.
   Jihye: I want to ask you if you have any dietary restrictions.
   Mrs. Lieberman: Well, I'm Jewish, so I'm not allowed to eat any pork or shellfish.
   Jihye: I'll let our dietitian know about your request.
   Mrs. Lieberman: Thank you very much. I was worried about the meals here.
   A: c) She can't eat shellfish and pork.
2. Dohyun: Good morning, Billy.
   Billy: Good morning, Ms. Dohyun.
   Dohyun: How are you feeling?
   Billy: I feel OK, but my stitches itch.
   Dohyun: That means you're healing well. The doctor will take out your stitches soon.
   Billy: Does it hurt when the doctor takes out the stitches?
   Dohyun: Just a tiny bit.
   A: d) He's worried it will hurt when the doctor takes out his stitches.
3. Hyoja: Mrs. Jennings, do you have any concerns about your hospital admission?
   Mrs. Jennings: I need to have heart surgery, and I'm worried about needing a blood transfusion.
   Hyoja: Well, there is some possibility you may need a tranfusion during surgery.
   Mrs. Jennings: I can't have a blood transfusion. I'm a Jehovah's Witness. Jehovah's Witnesses aren't allowed to have blood transfusions.
   Hyoja: I see. Why don't we talk about your wishes together with your husband and your doctor?
   A: c) Because of her religion.
4. Hyoja: Good morning. Mr. Philips. How are you feeling today?
   Mr. Philips: I'm feeling a lot of pain.
   Hyoja: I'm sorry to hear that. I'll talk to your doctor about increasing your painkillers.
   Mr. Philips: Thank you. I'd appreciate that.
   Hyoja: Do you have any other concerns or worries?
   Mr. Philips: Well, my cancer is getting worse. I'm worried about the pain. I'm afraid that my doctor won't give me enough painkillers.
   Hyoja: Please, don't worry about that. We'll do everything we can to keep you comfortable.
   A: a) He wants more painkillers.

Activity 3: Dialog (CD 32)

1. Welcome to this hospital
2. first visit
3. foreign patients
4. there are difference
5. special needs of
6. the main difference
7. The other thing
8. a person's religion
9. he'd be happy
10. nurse visiting from
11. Are you having any problems
12. I'm worried about
13. I can help explain
14. a chance to talk
15. didn't realize

Activity 4: Puzzle

1. c	6. b
2. b	7. b
3. a, b, c	8. b, c
4. c	9. c
5. a	10. c